Updates in Hallux Rigidus

Editor

JAMES A. NUNLEY II

FOOT AND ANKLE CLINICS

www.foot.theclinics.com

Consulting Editor
CESAR DE CESAR NETTO

September 2024 • Volume 29 • Number 3

ELSEVIER

1600 John F. Kennedy Boulevard • Suite 1800 • Philadelphia, Pennsylvania, 19103-2899

http://www.theclinics.com

FOOT AND ANKLE CLINICS Volume 29, Number 3
September 2024 ISSN 1083-7515, ISBN-978-0-443-13119-6

Editor: Megan Ashdown
Developmental Editor: Anita Chamoli

Foot and Ankle Clinics (ISSN 1083-7515) is published quarterly by Elsevier, Inc., 360 Park Avenue South, New York, NY 10010-1710. Months of issue are March, June, September, and December. Periodicals postage paid at New York, NY, and additional mailing offices. Subscription price per year is $369.00 (US individuals), $100.00 (US students), $397.00 (Canadian individuals), $100.00 (Canadian students), $514.00 (international individuals), and $215.00 (international students). For institutional access pricing please contact Customer Service via the contact information below.To receive student/resident rate, orders must be accompanied by name of affiliated institution, date of term, and the *signature* of program/residency coordinator on institution letterhead. Orders will be billed at individual rate until proof of status is received. Foreign air speed delivery is included in all *Clinics* subscription prices. All prices are subject to change without notice. Orders, claims, and journal inquiries: Please visit our Support Hub page https://service.elsevier.com for assistance.

Reprints. For copies of 100 or more, of articles in this publication, please contact the Commercial Reprints Department, Elsevier Inc., 360 Park Avenue South, New York, NY 10010-1710. Tel.: 212-633-3874; Fax: 212-633-3820; E-mail: reprints@elsevier.com.

CONSULTING EDITOR

Cesar de Cesar Netto, MD, PhD
Orthopaedic Foot and Ankle Surgeon
Associate Professor
Department of Orthopedic Surgery
Duke University
Durham, North Carolina, USA

EDITORIAL ADVISORY BOARD

Caio Augusto de Souza Nery, MD
Foot and Ankle Surgeon
Associate Professor
Orthopedic & Traumatology Department
Federal University of São Paulo
São Paulo, Brazil

Francois Lintz, MD, PhD
Orthopaedic Surgeon
Foot and Ankle Department
Ramsay Healthcare Clinique de l'Union
Saint Jean, France

Christopher D. Murawski, MD
Orthopedic Surgeon
Division of Foot and Ankle Surgery
Duke University
Durham, North Carolina, USA

Yoon-Chung Kim, MD, PhD
Associate Professor
Department of Orthopaedic Surgery
St. Vincent's Hospital
The Catholic University of Korea
Seoul, South Korea

Contributors

CONSULTING EDITOR

CESAR DE CESAR NETTO, MD, PhD
Orthopaedic Foot and Ankle Surgeon, Associate Professor, Department of Orthopedic Surgery, Duke University, Durham, North Carolina, USA

EDITOR

JAMES A. NUNLEY II, MD
J Leonard Goldner Endowed Professor, Goldner Jones Distinguished Professor, Division of Foot and Ankle Surgery, Department of Orthopaedic Surgery, Duke University, Durham, North Carolina, USA

AUTHORS

ANTOINE S. ACKER, MD
Research Scholar, Department of Orthopaedic Surgery, Duke University Medical Center, Durham, North Carolina, USA; Foot and Ankle Specialist, Centre of Foot and Ankle Surgery, Clinique La Colline, Geneva, Switzerland

ALBERT T. ANASTASIO, MD
Resident Physician, Department of Orthopaedics, Duke University Hospital, Durham, North Carolina, USA

ROBERT B. ANDERSON, MD
Orthopedist, Foot & Ankle Institute, OrthoCarolina, Charlotte, North Carolina, USA

ROHAN BHIMANI, MD, MBA
Fellow of Foot and Ankle Orthopaedic Surgery, Foot and Ankle Division, Department of Orthopaedic Surgery, Emory University School of Medicine, Emory Orthopedics, Atlanta, Georgia, USA

REBECCA CERRATO, MD
Orthopaedic Foot and Ankle Surgeon, Mercy Medical Center, The Institute for Foot and Ankle Reconstruction, Baltimore, Maryland, USA

CAROLINE CRISTOFARO, MBChB
Orthopaedic Resident, Department of Orthopaedics, University of Toronto, Department of Orthopaedics, St Michael's Hospital, Toronto, Ontario, Canada

TIMOTHY DANIELS, MD, FRCSC
Professor, Department of Orthopaedics, University of Toronto, Department of Orthopaedics, St Michael's Hospital, Toronto, Ontario, Canada

MARK E. EASLEY, MD
Associate Professor, Department of Orthopaedic Surgery, Duke University Medical Center, Duke University Hospital, Durham, North Carolina, USA

SCOTT J. ELLIS, MD
Associate Attending, Foot and Ankle Department, Weill Cornell Medical College, Hospital for Special Surgery, New York, New York, USA

AMANDA N. FLETCHER, MD, MSc
Orthopaedic Foot and Ankle Surgeon, OrthoCarolina, Charlotte, North Carolina, USA

GREGORY P. GUYTON, MD
Attending, Department of Orthopaedic Surgery, MedStar Union Memorial Hospital, Baltimore, Maryland, USA

MANSUR HALAI, BSc (Hons), MBChB, MRCS, FRCS (Tr & Orth)
Assistant Professor, Department of Orthopaedics, University of Toronto, Department of Orthopaedics, St Michael's Hospital, Toronto, Ontario, Canada

ANDREW E. HANSELMAN MD
Assistant Professor, Department of Orthopaedic Surgery, Duke University, Durham, North Carolina, USA

KENNETH J. HUNT, MD
Associate Professor, Foot and Ankle Surgery, Chief, Division of Foot and Ankle Surgery, Department of Orthopedic Surgery, University of Colorado, Aurora, Colorado, USA

MOHAMAD ISSA, MD
Foot and Ankle Orthopaedic Surgery Fellows, Department of Orthopaedic Surgery, Duke University Medical Center, Durham, North Carolina, USA

SAMEH A. LABIB, MD
Professor, Foot and Ankle Division, Department of Orthopaedic Surgery, Emory University School of Medicine, Emory Orthopedics, Atlanta, Georgia, USA

JEFFREY LILES, MD
Clinical Fellow, Department of Orthopaedic Surgery, Duke University Medical Center, Durham, North Carolina, USA

KEPLER ALENCAR MENDES DE CARVALHO, MD
Research Scholar, Department of Orthopaedic Surgery, Duke University, Durham, North Carolina, USA

RAMI MIZHER, MD
Research Assistant, Foot and Ankle Department, Hospital for Special Surgery, New York, USA

CHRISTOPHER D. MURAWSKI, MD
Orthopedist, Foot & Ankle Institute, OrthoCarolina, Charlotte, North Carolina, USA

JAMES A. NUNLEY II, MD
J Leonard Goldner Endowed Professor, Goldner Jones Distinguished Professor, Division of Foot and Ankle Surgery, Department of Orthopaedic Surgery, Duke University, Durham, North Carolina, USA

CONOR O'NEILL, MD
Foot and Ankle Orthopaedic Surgery Fellow, Department of Orthopaedic Surgery, Duke University Medical Center, Durham, North Carolina, USA

VANDAN PATEL, MD
Clinical Assistant Professor, Department of Orthopaedic Surgery, University of Michigan, Ann Arbor, Michigan, USA

LAVAN RAJAN, MD
Research Assistant, Foot and Ankle Department, Hospital for Special Surgery, New York, USA

SOLANGEL RODRIGUEZ-MATERON, MD
Fellow, Department of Orthopaedic Surgery, MedStar Union Memorial Hospital, Baltimore, Maryland, USA

KARL SCHWEITZER, MD
Foot and Ankle Orthopaedic Surgeon, Department of Orthopaedic Surgery, Duke University Medical Center, Durham, North Carolina, USA; Assistant Professor, Foot and Ankle, Raleigh, North Carolina, USA

AARON T. SCOTT, MD
Professor, Department of Orthopaedic Surgery, Wake Forest University School of Medicine, Winston-Salem, North Carolina, USA

ISABEL SHAFFREY, BS
Medical Student, Duke University School of Medicine, Durham, North Carolina, USA

YU MIN SUH, MD
Resident, Department of Orthopaedics, University of North Carolina at Chapel Hill, Chapel Hill, North Carolina, USA

JOSHUA N. TENNANT, MD
Associate Professor, Department of Orthopaedics, University of North Carolina at Chapel Hill, Chapel Hill, North Carolina, USA

BRADY T. WILLIAMS, MD
Orthopaedic Surgery Resident, Division of Foot and Ankle Surgery, Department of Orthopedic Surgery, University of Colorado, Aurora, Colorado, USA

COLLEEN WIXTED, MD
Resident Physician, Division of Foot and Ankle Surgery, Department of Orthopaedic Surgery, Duke University, Durham, North Carolina, USA

Contents

Hallux rigidus is a common degenerative condition of the hallux metatarso-phalangeal joint (MTPJ) characterized by pain, swelling, stiffness, and limited range of motion with characteristic corresponding clinical, physical examination, and radiographic findings. Many historical risks factors including trauma and family history and patient factors including hallux valgus interphalangeus and inflammatory arthropathies have a well-substantiated etiologic role in the disease process. The purpose of this section is to review the normal and pathologic anatomy and biomechanics of the hallux MTPJ while providing an overview of the current understanding and remain debate regarding the disease process.

The classification systems of hallux rigidus, including the Coughlin and Shurnas, Hattrup and Johnson, Regnauld, and Roukis classifications, allow for a comprehensive understanding of the condition's severity and aid in informed treatment decisions. The common techniques of radiological imaging, such as standard plain film radiographs, MRI, magnetic resonance arthrography computed tomography (CT), weightbearing CT, and ultrasound, which enable accurate assessment of joint degeneration and associated pathologies for optimal patient care, are reviewed.

Hallux rigidus is a degenerative arthritic condition affecting the first metatarsophalangeal joint. Prevalence in patients aged 50 years and above is estimated at 20% to 30%, with a portion being symptomatic. Conservative treatment's efficacy is linked to initial pain levels; though shoe modifications and insoles are commonly recommended, their true effectiveness lacks strong evidence. Injection therapy, including corticosteroids and hyaluronic acid, demonstrates varied outcomes, with about 50% of patients undergoing surgery within 1 to 2 years. The condition's etiology remains elusive, but recent biomechanical hypotheses hold promise.

Dorsal cheilectomy refers to a surgical resection of the dorsal osteophyte from the first metatarsal head. It is most often performed in patients with hallux rigidus, who have little to no midrange pain of the first metatarsophalangeal joint. The procedure is simple, quick, and maintains range of motion. Additional advantages of this procedure include low morbidity, quicker postoperative recovery, avoidance of costly implants, and the fact that the procedure does not inhibit future conversion to an arthrodesis. These proposed advantages have led some authors to advocate for the use of a cheilectomy, even in patients with more extensive disease.

Hallux rigidus represents the arthritis affecting the first metatarsophalangeal joint. It often leads to limited dorsiflexion, affecting gait and causing pain. Moberg osteotomy involves a dorsal closing wedge osteotomy on the proximal phalanx performed for early stages of hallux rigidus. This osteotomy shifts the load to the plantar aspect and compensates for the limited dorsiflexion. Moberg osteotomy can be combined with Akin osteotomy to create a biplanar correction for hallux interphalangeus. The procedure has favorable outcomes and high patient satisfaction rates with low complications. Larger high-quality studies are required to draw further on its benefits.

 Video content accompanies this article at http://www.foot.theclinics. com.

Interpositional arthroplasty for the treatment of hallux rigidus (HR) involves resection of the diseased joint surface and placement of spacer material within the joint to preserve length at the metatarsophalangeal joint while still allowing for range of motion. The majority of studies available in the literature have focused on capsular interpositional arthroplasty, revealing generally positive outcomes. Other forms of interpositional arthroplasty are less supported by long-term follow-up and large sample sizes. Moreover, there exists substantial heterogeneity in the studies evaluating interpositional arthroplasty. Despite the limitations of the current data, interpositional arthroplasty seems to be a viable treatment option for HR.

Hallux rigidus can present a difficult problem to both competitive and elite athletic populations. Once an appropriate diagnostic workup has been performed, nonoperative management strategies, including anti-inflammatory medications, injection therapies, shoewear modifications, and orthotic devices, represent the mainstay conservative management options. Surgical management can be considered where an athlete's athletic performance is limited. A joint-sparing cheilectomy can provide a predictable return to sport at the most elite levels. The addition of a proximal phalangeal osteotomy can be considered when necessary. Arthroplasty or arthrodesis techniques can be used for persistent symptoms or progressive disease, but with less predictable outcomes.

Hallux metatarsophalangeal joint cheilectomy is a joint-sparing technique that involves resection of the dorsal metatarsal head osteophytes; this may be achieved through minimally invasive and arthroscopic techniques. General indications for minimally invasive surgery (MIS) cheilectomy are mild-to-moderate hallux rigidus (Grades I–II) with symptomatic dorsal osteophytes causing dorsal impingement and/or shoe wear irritation in those who have failed extensive nonoperative management. The literature confirms equivalent outcomes to open cheilectomy; however, it is somewhat inconsistent regarding superiority. The theoretic benefits of MIS cheilectomy include better cosmesis, reduced wound complications, less soft tissue disruption, and faster recovery.

The Cartiva implant is a synthetic polyvinyl alcohol hydrogel cartilage substitute that is used as a treatment of first metatarsophalangeal joint arthritis. The implant was designed to relieve the pain associated with hallux rigidus while preserving or restoring range of motion. A summary of outcomes, reasons for these outcomes, and technique pearls will be reviewed here. Seminal articles and current evidence are all included in this article. The aim is for the surgeon to understand all the literature, allowing the surgeon to counsel their patients appropriately, optimize patient selection and to deal with complications.

 Video content accompanies this article at http://www.foot.theclinics.com.

First metatarsophalangeal joint (MTPJ) arthroplasty provides hallux rigidus patients with pain relief and preserved motion, offering an alternative to arthrodesis. Recent advancements in implant technology and surgical techniques have broadened treatment options. Although good outcomes have been documented in the literature, concerns persist regarding increased complications, uncertain long-term efficacy, and challenges in managing failed arthroplasties. Addressing bone loss resulting from the procedure further complicates salvage procedures. Larger cohorts and extended studies are necessary to establish efficacy of first MTPJ arthroplasty. Decisions must weigh the trade-offs between pain relief and potential complications, requiring thorough patient-surgeon discussions.

creates large osseous deficits and surgical management can be difficult. Salvage arthrodesis provides reliable joint stability while maintaining hallux length. Outcomes following conversion of a failed MTP joint arthroplasty to MTP joint arthrodesis have demonstrated consistent pain relief and high satisfaction: however, high rates of complication and nonunion have been reported. Bone graft may be necessary to fill large voids in the joint. Other revision options for failed arthroplasty have been described, but outcomes remain inconsistent and varied. Ultimately, conversion to MTP joint arthrodesis is the recommended intervention for treatment of the failed MTP arthroplasty implant, providing sufficient stability and pain relief.

FOOT AND ANKLE CLINICS

RELATED SERIES

Orthopedic Clinics
Clinics in Sports Medicine
Physical Medicine and Rehabilitation Clinics

THE CLINICS ARE NOW AVAILABLE ONLINE!
Access your subscription at:
www.theclinics.com

Preface

Hallux Rigidus Revisited

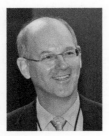

James A. Nunley, II, MD
Editor

It's been nearly 9 years since we published an issue about hallux rigidus in *Foot and Ankle Clinics of North America*, and the incidence of hallux rigidus has increased as our population ages. Over this time period there has been significant progress made in theories of etiology, pathology, classification schemes, surgical treatment, and results, all of which we have highlighted in this issue. I know in my own practice I have had to rethink my treatment algorithm based on much of the information included in this issue.

In this issue, I have called upon numerous experts with vast experience in the field to update us on these new findings, and I hope this information will be useful as you address your patients.

One special article that has been added to this issue is the treatment of hallux rigidus in the athlete. I am particularly grateful to Bob Anderson for sharing his experience, for as we know these athletes present their own special needs when confronted with significant pain and lack of function, yet they are still participating at the highest athletic levels.

MIS surgery is currently a hot topic in foot and ankle surgery, and we have updated not only the surgical techniques but also the results of current literature relating to MIS surgery.

The use of hydrogel implants has garnered much recent attention, and this issue expands upon the advocates as well as the detractors of this procedure.

Foot Ankle Clin N Am 29 (2024) xv–xvi
https://doi.org/10.1016/j.fcl.2024.03.001
1083-7515/24/© 2024 Elsevier Inc. All rights reserved.

foot.theclinics.com

As with all literature, our knowledge continues to expand over previous literature, so I hope this issue will prove useful as we address an increase in the incidence of hallux rigidus in our aging population.

James A. Nunley II, MD
Goldner Jones Distinguished Professor of Orthopaedic Surgery
Duke University
Durham, NC, USA

E-mail address:
James.nunley@duke.edu

Hallux Rigidus
Anatomy and Pathology

Brady T. Williams, MD, Kenneth J. Hunt, MD*

KEYWORDS

- Hallux rigidus • Forefoot arthritis • Metatarsus primus elevatus • Hallux limitus

KEY POINTS

- The hallux metatarsophalangeal joint (MTPJ) is an intricate anatomic complex that facilitates well-coordinated movements throughout gait and athletic activities.
- The hallux MTPJ is the most common location of arthritis in the foot and ankle, and second most common in the lower extremity, second only to the knee.
- The clinical presentation of hallux rigidus is consistent in the literature including stiffness, pain, locking, cosmetic swelling, altered (supinated) gait, inability to rise up on the toe, painful dorsal bump, and hallux MTPJ pain with radiographic evidence of flattening of the metatarsal head, loss of joint space, and dorsal osteophytes.
- Predisposing patient factors and clinical findings include trauma, family history, inflammatory arthropathy, flattened or chevron metatarsal head morphology, presence of osteochondral lesions, and hallux valgus interphalangeus.
- Other factors, including first ray hypermobility, pes planus, equinus contracture, metatarsal length, metatarsus adductus, equinus contracture, flexor hallucis longus pathology, and metatarsus primus elevatus, remain topics of debate.

INTRODUCTION

Hallux rigidus, a Latin phrase translating as "stiff big toe" is a progressive condition of the hallux metatarsophalangeal joint (MTPJ) characterized by pain, stiffness, loss of motion, and joint degeneration. The condition was first described by Davis-Colley in the late 1800s, initially termed "hallucis flexus."[1] In short succession, Cotterill coined the currently used term, "hallux rigidus."[2,3] Since its original descriptions, hallux rigidus has been a topic of significant focus in the foot and ankle literature including anatomic, radiographic, biomechanical and kinematic descriptions to better elucidate the cause and pathogenesis of the disease process. Findings have aided in the development of nonoperative treatments and surgical interventions that have been studied with outcomes-based studies to identify optimal treatment strategies. The purpose of

Division of Foot and Ankle Surgery, Department of Orthopedic Surgery, University of Colorado, 12631 East 17th Avenue, Room 4508, Aurora, CO 80045, USA
* Corresponding author.
E-mail address: Kenneth.j.hunt@cuanschutz.edu

Foot Ankle Clin N Am 29 (2024) 371–387
https://doi.org/10.1016/j.fcl.2023.12.002
1083-7515/24/© 2024 Elsevier Inc. All rights reserved.

foot.theclinics.com

this section is to summarize the normal anatomy and biomechanics of the hallux MTPJ, and the pathologic progression of hallux rigidus within the context of patient factors and the current literature.

ANATOMY

The hallux MTPJ is a complex condyloid articulation, previously described as a hammock within which the metatarsal head sits.[4] It is composed of the hallux metatarsal head, proximal phalanx base, 2 sesamoids, flexor and extensor tendons, and the supporting capsuloligamentous structures that collectively facilitate flexion, extension, abduction, adduction, and circumduction (**Figs. 1** and **2**). A comprehensive understanding of the normal anatomy is crucial to clinical evaluation, diagnosis, development of treatment algorithms, and overall understanding of pathogenesis.

The hallux metatarsal head has a large convex asymmetric articular surface, with a smaller radius of curvature in the sagittal plane than in the transverse plane, which contrasts the lesser metatarsals.[5] Although contiguous, the articular surface can be functionally divided into superior and inferior segments. The dorsal segment articulates with the proximal phalanx, sloping dorsally and posteriorly before blending with the metaphysis of the metatarsal shaft. The inferior segment articulates plantarly with the sesamoids and is further divided by a ridge into medial (tibial) and lateral (fibular) articulations with defined grooves for the corresponding sesamoids. The proximal phalanx base has a concave articular surface, relatively smaller compared with the metatarsal head, again with a radius of curvature that is smaller in the sagittal than in the transverse plane. Adjacent to the articular surface lie bony prominences that correspond to attachments for the extensor hallucis brevis (EHB), flexor hallucis brevis (FHB), adductor hallucis, and abductor hallucis. The hallux MTPJ joint is circumferentially enveloped by the joint capsule, which in neutral flexion, seems thickened and redundant at the metatarsal neck attachment.[6]

Plantarly, the medial (tibial) and lateral (fibular) sesamoids are embedded within the plantar plate construct, articulating in the corresponding grooves of the plantar metatarsal head that serve as a fulcrum during propulsive gait.[7] The sesamoids arise from multiple ossification centers, which typically being ossifying around the age of 8 years[8] (see **Fig. 2**). The tibial sesamoid is larger, more ovoid in shape, and typically more distal within the plantar plate, whereas the fibular sesamoid is smaller and more round.[7,9] Up to one-third of sesamoids are bipartite (4%–35%), most commonly the

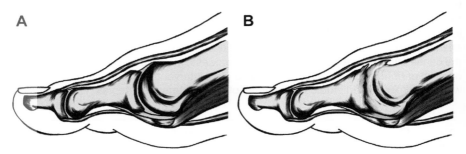

A   **B**

Fig. 1. Reproduced with permission from Lucas and Hunt 2015.[82] (*A*) Sagittal illustration of normal hallux MTPJ anatomy. (*B*) Sagittal illustration of the characteristic hallux rigidus pathologic condition including dorsal osteophyte formation, narrowing of the joint space, and flattening of the metatarsal head. (*Courtesy of* Nathan T. Formaini, DO, Holy Cross Orthopedic Institute, Fort Lauderdale, FL.)

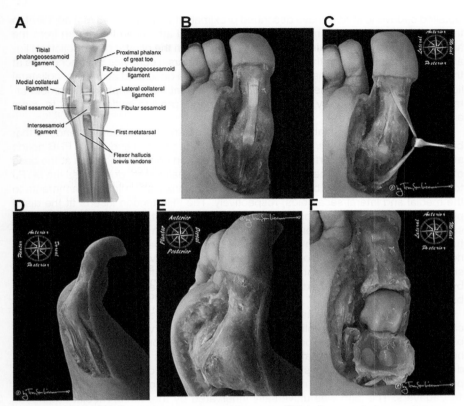

Fig. 2. Reproduced with permission from Waldrop 2021.[83] (*A*) Illustrated plantar plate anatomy of the first MTP joint. (*B*) Cadaveric plantar anatomy of the first MTP joint with the FHL intact and (*C*) retracted medially. (*D, E*) Lateral view. (*F*) Plantar view with the plantar plate reflect from the proximal phalanx revealing the plantar metatarsal head and sesamoids imbedded in the plantar structures. (*From* Clanton TO, Waldrop NE. Athletic injuries to the soft tissues of the foot and ankle. In: Coughlin MJ, Saltzman CL, Anderson RB, eds. Mann's Surgery of the Foot and Ankle. 9th ed. Philadelphia, PA: Elsevier Saunders; 2014: 1531-1687; with permission. Illustrated by Andy Evansen.)

tibial sesamoid, and can frequently bilateral occurrence.[8,9] The sesamoids also have numerous capsuloligamentous attachments integral to function and stability of the hallux MTPJ. The sesamoids are imbedded within a capsuloligamentous complex and are tethered together by the intersesamoid ligament, which serves as an indirect bridge connecting the FHB, adductor hallucis, and abductor hallucis, and are confluent with the synovial sheath of the flexor hallucis longus (FHL).[6,7] The sesamoids are further tethered to the metatarsal head and proximal phalanx base through the metatarsal sesamoid and sesamoid phalangeal ligaments, the latter of which are thicker, restrain proximal migration, and are more commonly injured in hyperextension injuries.[6,7,10] The sesamoids are furthermore enveloped in the capsuloligamentous or hallucal sesamoid complex, more commonly referred to as the plantar plate.

The plantar plate has significant biomechanical contributions to the stability and function of the MTPJ joint including dispersing body weight across the sesamoids and protecting the articular surface. The plantar plate complex receives contributions from osseous, capsular, fibrocartilaginous, ligamentous, and tendinous structures.[6,7]

Detailed cadaveric studies have described proximal attachments 1.73 mm adjacent to the articular margin of the metatarsal head and distal attachments 0.3 mm from the articular margin on the proximal phalanx.[7] Distinct from the plantar plate, collateral ligaments run obliquely from the tubercles on the metatarsal condyles to attachments at the base of the proximal phalanx.[6] Other authors have described accessory collateral ligaments with capsular, metatarsal sesamoid ligament, and peripheral sesamoid attachments.[11,12] Collectively, the collateral ligaments provide static stability to varus and valgus stress.

Mobility and dynamic stability of the MTPJ is conferred by numerous tendons that both cross and insert at the hallux MTPJ. Plantarly, the medial and lateral FHB heads attach along the plantar surfaces of the sesamoids and continue to attach at the base of the proximal phalanx. The adductor and abductor hallucis tendons cross the MTPJ to their attachments at the base of the proximal phalanx with variable attachments to the medial and lateral sesamoids, respectively. The FHL tendon inserts at the distal phalanx, passing through a fibrous sheath at the MTPJ that is confluent with the inter-sesamoid ligament.[6] Proximally, the FHL courses through a fibro-osseous tunnel at the posteromedial ankle often accompanied by muscle fibers.[13] Compression or stenosis can occur at this location leading to stenosing synovitis, which has a hypothesized role in the development of hallux rigidus.[13,14] Dorsally, extension is facilitated by the complex of EHB and extensor hallucis longus (EHL), extensor hood, and sagittal bands.[6]

The neuroanatomy of the hallux MTPJ joint has also been well characterized. This carries pathoanatomical implications with respect to nerve compression by dorsal osteophytes. Furthermore, understanding the innervations of the hallux MTPJ is necessary for performing safe surgical approaches, as well as guiding possible denervation procedures for symptomatic relief. Çatal and colleagues reported the proportion of hallux MTPJs innervated by specific sensory nerves in a sample of 14 cadavers. The joint was universally innervated by the dorsal medial cutaneous nerve, with varying innervations of the deep peroneal (11 out of 14), medial hallucal (6 out of 14), and lateral hallucal nerves (5 out of 14).[15] This is observed clinically with patients commonly presenting with dysesthesias of the dorsomedial cutaneous nerve.[9]

BIOMECHANICS

Both normal and pathologic biomechanics and kinematics of the hallux have been well characterized. The first ray is a crucial component of the medial column and acts as a rigid lever during heel rise. During gait, the first ray is the most heavily loaded, bearing 119% of the body weight with approximately 90% of ground reactive forces being transferred through the MTPJ with peak forces of 600 N documented in healthy subjects.[16–18] The sesamoids transmit approximately 50% of body weight during push off and up to 300% in higher demand activities.[11] The normal hallux MTPJ has impressive flexibility in the sagittal plane while also allowing transverse plane motion. On average, controls demonstrate a total sagittal arc of 100° to 130°, with 30° to 40° of plantarflexion and 60° to 90° of dorsiflexion, which can be assessed with Buell (non–weight-bearing), Dananberg (simulated weight-bearing), and Jack (weight-bearing) tests.[9,19,20] Normative values for these states have been reported to be 82°, 60°, and 40°, respectively.[20,21] The degree of maximal dorsiflexion during gait depends on footwear, with 60° reported when bare foot, 45° to 50° in soft shoes, and 25° to 30° in stiff shoes.[22] In the transverse plane, studies demonstrate an arc of motion equivalent to 15% of the metatarsal head.[19] However, static measurements at extremes of motion have not correlated well with function; therefore, authors have developed measures of joint flexibility with descriptive parameters including early flexibility (first 25% of motion), laxity angle, and torque angle (torque and angle at the intersection of tangent lines at early and late flexibility on torque-angle curve).[23,24]

Throughout the gait cycle, there are 2 episodes of dorsiflexion observed at the hallux MTPJ throughout the stance phase. The first is at heel strike and the second is at toe off and heel rise. During this, the proximal phalanx glides on the metatarsal head with compressive forces noted dorsally near the end of dorsiflexion.[19] The ability to maintain passive dorsiflexion during the second half of gait likely minimizes dorsal compressive forces, thereby providing rationale for the implication of FHL stenosis, reduced excursion, and resistance to dorsiflexion in the pathogenesis of hallux rigidus.[14,25] In hallux rigidus, restricted motion is observed in both planes with a total sagittal arc of 69°, 49° of dorsiflexion, and a 50% reduction in transverse plane motion relative to controls.[19] However, dynamic radiographic studies indicate clinical measurements may underestimate range of motion, particularly in more severe disease (<30° of clinically measured dorsiflexion) due to questionable reliability of widely used goniometric measurements.[24,26] Other metrics, including laxity angle, are significantly reduced relative to controls when controlling for age.[23,24]

At the joint, restricted dorsiflexion by periarticular osteophytes, results in displaced, eccentric, and variable joint centers of rotation with random surface velocity vectors, indicating abnormal jamming of joint surfaces throughout the arc of motion.[19] Through gait analysis, numerous alterations from normal patterns have been described. Betts and colleagues demonstrated increased great toe pressures, shorter stride length, decreased dorsiflexion, and early toe off.[27] Canseco and colleagues demonstrated prolonged stance phase in a sample of 22 hallux rigidus patients compared with controls with subsequent improvement in walking speed, cadence, stride length, and stance/swing phase ratio following cheilectomy.[28,29] Cansel and colleagues reported inversion and supination of the forefoot and hindfoot in attempts to offload the hallux, resulting in transfer of load to the lesser metatarsals and upstream limb effects including shorter stride length, higher ankle dorsiflexion, and compensatory pelvic rotation.[30] Other pathologic processes, just as adjacent joint disease including ankle arthritis, have been shown to alter mechanics at the MTPJ, including increase forefoot eversion and valgus shift of the hallux, and decreased push off strength.[28,29]

The pathomechanics of hallux rigidus have been used to rationalize orthotics and shoe wear modifications. Instruments are aimed at symptoms reductions including limiting irritation of dorsal osteophytes through high and broad toe box shoes, reducing motion of the hallux MTPJ through rigid orthotics, and limiting mechanical stress and decompressing the dorsal joint, by raising the first metatarsal to allow for plantarflexion of the proximal phalanx and unloading the medial column in settings of increased pronation.[31,32]

HALLUX RIGIDUS
Incidence and Epidemiology

The hallux MTPJ is the most common location of arthritis in the foot and ankle, and second most common in the lower extremity, second only to the knee.[9,33,34] Collectively, this has a significant impact on patients, and society, with affected individuals reporting lower SF-36 physical and social subscales.[35] Prevalence of symptomatic hallux rigidus ranges from 2.5% to 10% in adults.[36–38] However, radiographic assessment does suggest a predictable increase with age including a 10% prevalence of radiographic disease in patients aged 20 to 34 years, 20% to 48% in adults aged older than 40 years, and 77% in patients aged older than 80 years.[34,39–41] In a large series of hallux rigidus patients from a single institution, the average age of onset was 43 years (range 13–70), with 67% of patients reporting a family history.[42] Although initial presentation was typically unilateral (81%), the majority of patients (79%) developed or reported bilateral disease over a mean follow-up of 8.9 years.[42] Historically, bilateral disease has been considered almost universal in patients with a significant family history (95%); however, family history has not been correlated with age of onset. In contrast, unilateral disease has typically correlated with reported trauma; however, Coughlin and Shurnas did not find this association to be statistically significant.[42] Studies historically have also reported a female predilection; however, this has not been consistently confirmed in the subsequent literature.[37,41,42]

Clinical History and Examination

Clinically, hallux rigidus presents with a consistent constellation of symptoms including joint stiffness (**Fig. 3**), pain with joint motion, soft tissue swelling, and shoe wear intolerance.[42,43] Patients commonly present with osteophyte formation on the dorsal aspect of the distal metatarsal head and proximal aspect of the proximal phalanx.[38,42] The predominant complaints of patients are centered on pain, limited range of motion, and pain with extremes of motion due to impingement of dorsal osteophytes with terminal dorsiflexion, and stretch of the EHL over dorsal osteophytes at terminal plantarflexion.[9] Early in the disease process, motion limitations preferentially

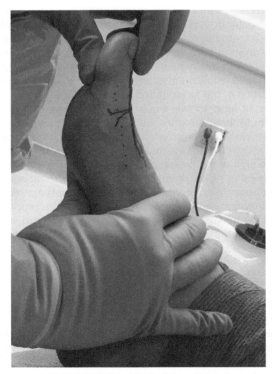

Fig. 3. Clinical photograph demonstrating physical examination under anesthesia demonstrating characteristic findings of hallux rigidus with significantly limited passive dorsiflexion.

affect dorsiflexion, altering regular gait mechanics and the ability to push off. As the disease process progresses and cartilage is worn centrally, patients eventually develop pain during midrange of motion due to advanced osteoarthritis as indicated by the "grind test." Dorsal prominences themselves, can also be a direct source of pain, interacting with more constrictive show wear and irritating the traversing dorsal cutaneous nerve.[9]

Aside from patient-reported symptoms, several commonalities on physical examination can be observed by a clinician stiffness, pain, locking, cosmetic swelling, altered (supinated) gait, inability to rise up on the toe, painful dorsal bump, and MTPJ pain.[42] Collectively, range or motion, radiographic findings, and clinical features have been used for the development of a variety of classification systems.[38]

Patient history

Despite the long-standing recognition of the pathologic condition, the cause of hallux rigidus still remains a source of debate, with many cases deemed to be idiopathic.[36,42] Patient factors and history, predominantly injury, trauma, and family history have been a focus of discussion. Coughlin and Shurnas reported a family history in 67% of patients overall, and 95% in patients with bilateral disease.[42] However, they did not find that family history correlated with age of onset or disease severity. Singular traumatic injury and repetitive microtrauma have been put forth as risk factors.[38,43,44] Repetitive or singular traumatic injury are thought to be the most common cause of hallux rigidus, particularly in unilateral disease.[43–45] However, this has not been consistently supported.[38,42] In the sample presented by Coughlin and Shurnas, acute trauma was reported in adolescent idiopathic disease, with 78% of patients with unilateral disease reporting a history of trauma.[42] However, others report only 14% of patients with a recalled history of trauma, although this is often clouded by delayed degenerative sequelae of trauma and recall bias.[46] This in part led to lending credence to the concept of repetitive microtrauma, perhaps related to hypermobility, initially discussed by Jack in 1940.[47]

Clinical and radiographic risk factors

A variety of patient factors, physical examination findings, and concurrent pathology have been implicated in the risk for developing hallux rigidus. However, there remains significant debate regarding the correlated and causative factors. Several clinical factors and imaging correlates have associated with hallux rigidus. Clinical features include first ray hypermobility,[47,48] gastrocnemius equinus and Achilles contracture,[48] forefoot pronation or pes planus,[48–50] hallux valgus,[48,51,52] hallux valgus interphalangeus (HVI),[42,48,53] pathologic limitations in FHL excursion,[14] adjacent joint or other foot and ankle arthroses,[54] inflammatory arthropathies,[54] and foot wear.[32] Although radiographic parameters have included flat or chevron metatarsal head morphology,[42,43,53,55] osteochondritis dissecans,[44,52,56] long or short first metatarsal,[46,57–60] metatarsus primus elevatus (MPE),[42,45,61–63] and metatarsus adductus.[42]

First ray hypermobility

Hypermobility of the first ray was discussed by Morton in 1928 and further discussed as a contributor to hallux rigidus by Jack in 1940.[47,64] Measurements were subsequently described by Klaue and colleagues.[65] However, this has not been subsequently demonstrated clinically, with some publishing contradictory data. In a small sample of 7 hallux rigidus patients, Coughlin and Shurnas did not report any patients with first ray hypermobility, which was further supported in a larger series of 110 patients.[38,66] Greisberg and colleagues measured first metatarsal translation in 345 feet (315 patients) with varying first ray pathologic conditions, demonstrating decreased mobility and elevation of the first ray in hallux rigidus compared with those with other medial column pathologic condition.[67]

Equinus contracture and pes planus

Gastrocnemius or Achilles contracture and pes planus have been suggested contributors to the development of hallux rigidus.[48–50] However, Coughlin and Shurnas specifically investigated this using Harris matt evaluation, reporting no correlation of hallux rigidus and pes planus or gastrocnemius contracture compared with historical data.[66,68] In another large study of 110 patient with hallux rigidus, Coughlin and Shurnas reported no difference in equinus contracture rates compared with the general population, and only an 11% rate in pes planus.[38,42]

Hallux valgus and hallux valgus interphalangeus

Several authors have identified a correlation between HVI (**Fig. 4**) and hallux rigidus with both clinical and radiographic assessments of hallux rigidus.[42,48,53,69] It is thought that HVI may predisposed patients to the development of hallux rigidus due to resultant stiffness of the hallux MTPJ through resistance of transverse plane motion.[42] Hypermobility of the interphalangeal joint has been thought to become deformed and degenerative over time.[48] As such, proximal phalanx osteotomies have been described for early disease.[53] In contrast, correlations with hallux valgus have not been well established in the literature despite early observations.[48,51,52] Coughlin and Shurnas only reported a 12% (15 out of 127 feet) rate of concurrent radiographic hallux valgus and hallux rigidus, with only 2 symptomatic feet.[42]

Flexor hallucis longus contracture/stenosis

The FHL acts late in stance phase to plantarflex the hallux MTPJ and secondarily plantarflex the ankle, counteracting ground reactive forces and stabilizing the medial longitudinal arch.[18] Reduced excursion of the FHL has been proposed to play a role in the development of disease. This is based on extrapolation of the clinical condition known as functional hallux limitus in which decreased range of motion is observed with weight-bearing in the absence of degenerative changes.[9] Hintermann and colleagues demonstrated the FHL has approximately 27 mm of excursion during passive ankle

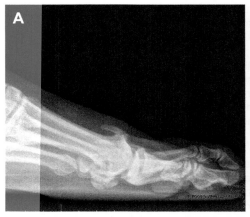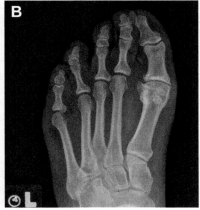

Fig. 4. Representative weight-bearing radiographs of a left foot (Male, 52 years) including the (A) lateral view demonstrating characteristic dorsal osteophytes of the distal metatarsal and proximal phalanx on the lateral view, with additional evidence on the (B) anteroposterior view of HVI (approximately 18°).

and hindfoot motion.[70] Contracture or stenosis, typically at the fibro-osseous tunnel in the posteromedial ankle, because of a forceful plantarflexion injury can lead to triggering of the great toe joints and decrease the efficiency of body weight transfer during heel-off. Downstream, this can result in eccentric rotation of the proximal phalanx on the metatarsal head, dorsal impingement, and arthritis changes.[14,21,25]

In a subset of 10 patients with FHL tenosynovitis and reduced MTP dorsiflexion, Michelson and colleagues reported relief of pain with treatment of the tenosynovitis.[25] In a cadaveric study, Kirane and colleagues measured FHL forces and excursion, first metatarsal forces, and first MTPJ forces in a simulated gait cycle with different degrees of FHL stenosis at 2, 4, and 6 mm proximal to the joint.[14] Authors demonstrated peak FHL tension during 70% to 85% of the stance phase, dorsally directed joint reactive forces with the onset of dorsiflexion (50% of stance phase), which were positively correlated with FHL tension. Authors concluded that simulated stenosis resulted in increased dorsally directed joint reactive forces early in the gait cycle, which supports FHL pathologic condition as a possible predisposing cause of hallux rigidus.[14]

Inflammatory arthropathies and adjacent joint disease
Systemic inflammatory arthropathies and adjacent joint arthrosis has also been correlated with hallux rigidus. Bejarano-Pineda and colleagues compared rates of hallux rigidus between the general population and those with end-stage ipsilateral ankle arthritis undergoing total ankle arthroplasty.[54] In 870 feet (809 patients, mean age 62.5 ± 10.5 years, 50.4% men), there was a significantly higher rate (72.9%) of hallux rigidus compared with the general population. This trend increased with age with a 47.6% prevalence in patients aged younger than 40 years and 92.6% in patients aged older than 80 years, supporting the additive effects of altered mechanics. The connection between hallux rigidus and inflammatory arthropathies such as rheumatoid, seronegative arthropathies, and gout has been well documented.[54]

Imaging

Radiographic evaluation is a uniform component of the initial evaluation of hallux rigidus. Typical findings of disease, as summarized by Coughlin and Shurnas in their review of the literature, include osteophyte formation, loose bodies, subchondral sclerosis, widening and flattening of the metatarsal head, and joint space narrowing[42] (**Fig. 5**). These findings are universally accepted as consequences of the disease process. However, other correlated radiographic findings are still debated in their classification as causative factors or resultant features of the disease process, including metatarsal articular morphology,[42,43,53,55] osteochondritis dissecans,[44,52] long or short first metatarsal,[46,57–60] and metatarsus adductus[42] and MPE.[42,45,61–63]

Metatarsal head morphology
The shape and congruity of the metatarsal head has been previously correlated with prevalence of disease.[42,43,53,55] Specifically, a flattened or chevron-shaped metatarsal head has been associated with hallux rigidus in multiple prior studies. Coughlin and Shurnas[42] and Hunt and Anderson,[53] in reports on patients with hallux rigidus, reported a 73% and 79% rates, respectively of flattened, squared, or chevron-shaped metatarsal head in patients with hallux rigidus.[42,53] Cadaveric investigations have also corroborated this, reported larger measured radius of curvature in hallux rigidus specimens.[55]

Osteochondritis dissecans and osteochondral lesions
Presence of osteochondritis dissecans (OCD) or other osteochondral lesions (**Fig. 6**) have been proposed as a risk factor and possible precursor to the development of hallux rigidus due to their frequent occurrence in these patients.[44,52] Goodfellow

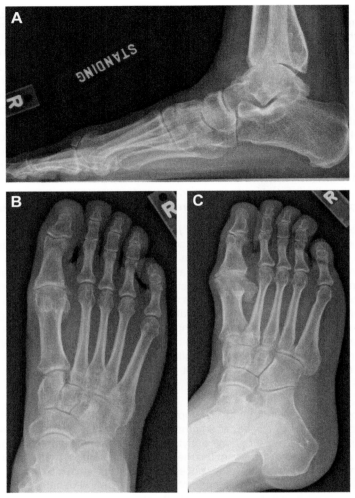

Fig. 5. Three weight-bearing views of a right foot (Male, 38 years) including (*A*) lateral view with evidence of dorsal osteophytes of the distal metatarsal and proximal phalanx. In addition, there is evidence of hallux metatarsus elevatus (8.7 mm) with concurrent tibiotalar arthritis. (*B*) Anteroposterior and (*C*) oblique views demonstrate characteristic loss of joint space, subchondral sclerosis, and periarticular osteophytes.

proposed that OCD lesions may progress to subsequent flattening of the metatarsal head that is seen in the progression of hallux rigidus.[56] McMaster reported 100% of young patients (mean age 21 years) were found to have OCD lesions on radiographs that uniformly correlated with an identifiable episode of trauma.[44]

Metatarsal length
Abnormal length of the first metatarsal, either long or short, has been theorized to play a role in the development of hallux rigidus and used for the rationale of various shortening osteotomies.[3,46,57–60] Historically, authors have hypothesized that prolonged presence of the distal metatarsal epiphysis results in a longer first metatarsal and overloading of the hallux MTPJ.[71] Coughlin and Shurnas reported no difference in rates of

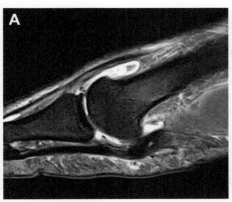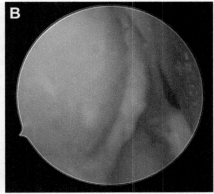

Fig. 6. Representative magnetic resonance and arthroscopic images of a left hallux (Female, 47 years) including a (A) Sagittal fat-suppressed proton density sequence demonstrating a large full thickness cartilage defect of the distal metatarsal head with multiple loose bodies, effusion, and synovitis. (B) Intraoperative arthroscopic image demonstrating full thickness cartilage lesion of the dorsal/central metatarsal head with exposed subchondral bone.

long first metatarsal compared with those of the general population.[42] In contrast, Calvo and colleagues published a case control study of 132 surgically feet with hallux rigidus (72 patients) and 132 control feet (66 volunteers), reporting a greater mean first metatarsal length in patients compared with that of controls.[58] The significance metatarsal length and rationale for various metatarsal osteotomies remains debated.

Metatarsus adductus
Coughlin and Shurnas reported 35 patients with metatarsus adductus (31.8%). Although more common in patients with hallux rigidus than the general population, no clear correlative or causative relationship has been established.[42]

Metatarsus primus elevatus
Elevation of the hallux on weight-bearing radiographs, or Metatarsus Primus Elevatus was initially described in a single case by Lambrinudi in 1938 and suggested as a cause of hallux rigidus.[61] In addition to the technique described by Lambrinudi, various plantarflexion osteotomies to address MPE have been subsequently described, including the Wilson, Austin bunionectomy, Youngswick, Watermann, and other basilar osteotomies.[46,51,61,72–74] However, studies have also demonstrated that MPE improves with surgical intervention, even when a plantarflexion metatarsal osteotomy is not performed.[38,66] Despite some proposing surgical correction, it remains unclear whether MPE is a cause or a consequence of disease. Multiple authors have argued a range of MPE to be a normal variant, with multiple radiographic studies demonstrating no significant differences between patients and controls.[45,62,69]

Given the overlap of patients and controls, there have been attempts to establish new measurement techniques and threshold values of pathologic MPE, ranging from 5 to 8 mm, to serve as diagnostic tools.[38,42,45,75] In a study comparing patients with hallux rigidus with asymptomatic controls and patients with Morton neuroma, Horton and colleagues reported no significant differences in MPE in patients with hallux rigidus (7.8 mm vs 7.9 vs 7.9).[45] However, authors did report slightly higher MPE measurements in advanced disease (Grade III: 9.2 mm; Grade II: 7.4 mm; and Grade I: 7.3 mm). Similarly, Coughlin and Shurnas reported a mean MPE of 5.5 mm in a sample of 110 patients and deemed this to be within normal anatomic variability.[42]

Subsequently, Bouchaicha and colleagues published on 295 randomly selected feet (221 patients, mean age 54 years), 99 with hallux rigidus, 99 with hallux valgus, and 97 with normal radiographic hallux MTPJs, reporting significant higher MPE in patients with hallux rigidus (5.2 mm) compared with patients with hallux valgus (2.8 mm) and controls (2.6 mm).[75] Jones and colleagues compared 65 patients with hallux rigidus with 65 size-matched controls, using 3 previously established and 4 newly described measurements,[45,75–77] including first metatarsal uncoverage angle, first metatarsal midpoint uncoverage angle, first metatarsal longitudinal axis uncoverage angle, and proximal phalanx-first metatarsal angle. All newly described measurements were correlated with hallux rigidus.[76] Most recently, Anwander and colleagues published a retrospective case control series of 50 patients including 25 with hallux rigidus, demonstrating a higher mean elevation (8.3 ± 1.7 mm) compared with that of controls (3.0 ± 2 mm), greater lateral first-second intermetatarsal angle (IMA; 3.6 ± 2.5 vs −0.7 ± 2.8), with no significant difference in first metatarsal declination angle. However, only 60% of hallux rigidus patients were determined to have MPE (compared with 0 controls).[78] These conflicting results from these studies are further clouded by the inherent limitations of plain radiographs.

Weight-bearing computed tomography
Historically, measurements on conventional radiographs have presented inherent limitations because of projection ankle and overlapping metatarsals. Since its advent and increasing availability, weight-bearing computed tomography (WBCT) has been used to more accurately assess many previously described radiographic measures and their association with hallux rigidus. Cheung and colleagues compared 50 controls and 50 patients with symptomatic hallux rigidus first and second metatarsal declination angles, first and second metatarsal lengths, first to second IMA, hallux valgus angle (HVA), and foot width, demonstrating the presence of MPE in patients with hallux rigidus, with greater MPE in more advanced disease.[79] Lee and colleagues compared samples of hallux valgus (27), hallux rigidus (26), and asymptomatic controls (30) with respect to measures of instability, including first tarsometatarsal (TMT) angle, dorsal translation of the first metatarsal at the first TMT joint, plantar distance between the medial cuneiform and first metatarsal in the sagittal plane, HVA, intermetatarsal angle (IMA), and rotational profiles of the medial cuneiform in the coronal plane. Authors reported increased dorsal translation of the first metatarsal and increased plantar distance between the medial cuneiform and the first metatarsal in both hallux valgus and hallux rigidus compared with controls, possibly lending credence to earlier hypothesis of sagittal first ray instability historically suggested by Morton and Jack.[47,64,80] In a similar study of 30 feet with hallux rigidus and 30 controls, Lee and colleagues compared HVA, MPE, first metatarsal declination angle, and first-second metatarsal declination ratio. All indicators of MPE were increased in patients with hallux rigidus including increased HVA and MPE, decreased first metatarsal declination (declination angle and first-second ratio), with 70% of patients with hallux rigidus demonstrating dorsal translation (step off) of the first TMT joint.[81–83] In contrast, no significant difference was observed in metatarsal length or forefoot adduction and supination. The authors furthermore proposed a WBCT threshold of 4.19 mm of MPE for the diagnosis of hallux rigidus with 77% sensitivity. As WBCT becomes more ubiquitous, earlier debates regarding plain radiographic measurement may gain more clarity and move closer to consensus.

SUMMARY

The anatomy of the hallux MTP is an intricate complex that facilitates well-coordinated movements throughout gait and athletic activities. Although the signs, symptoms, and presentation of hallux rigidus are nearly universally recognized, significant debate remains as to the specific cause and causative risk factors of disease development. The presentation of hallux rigidus is consistent in the literature including pain, swelling, limited range of motion asymmetrically affecting dorsiflexion, and dorsal osteophytes. Radiographically, this presents with flattening of the metatarsal head, loss of joint space, and dorsal osteophytes. Predisposing patient historical factors including trauma and family history are frequently present, correlating with unilateral and bilateral disease, respectively. Clinical and radiographic findings, including inflammatory arthropathy, flattened or chevron metatarsal head morphology, presence of osteochondral lesions, and HVI, seem to have general acceptance of correlation with disease. However, other factors, including first ray hypermobility, pes planus, equinus contracture, metatarsal length, metatarsus adductus, equinus contracture, FHL pathologic condition, and MPE remain topics of debate that perhaps will be better elucidated with emerging technologies such as WBCT.

CLINICS CARE POINTS

- The hallux MTPJ is the most common location of arthritis in the foot and ankle that reliably increases with age.
- Hallux rigidus has a relatively consistent clinical presentation including stiffness asymmetrically affect dorsiflexion, pain, locking, cosmetic swelling, altered (supinated) gait, painful dorsal bump, and hallux MTPJ pain.
- Standard weight-bearing radiographs regularly demonstrate flattening of the metatarsal head, loss of joint space, and dorsal osteophytes.
- Predisposing patient factors and clinical findings with reasonable consensus and current evidence include earlier trauma (single episode, repetitive, or iatrogenic), family history (often with bilateral disease), inflammatory arthropathy, flattened or chevron metatarsal head morphology, presence of osteochondritis dissecans or osteochondral lesions, and HVI.
- Clinical and radiographic findings that current have insufficient evidence or remain a topic of debate include first ray hypermobility, pes planus, equinus contracture, metatarsal length, metatarsus adductus, equinus contracture, FHL pathologic condition, and MPE.

DISCLOSURE

The authors have no pertinent financial or funding disclosures related to the content of this article.

REFERENCES

1. Davis-Colley N. Contraction of the metatarsophalangeal joint of the great toe (hallux flexus). Br Med J 1887;1:728.
2. Cotterill JM. The pathology of hallux rigidus. Br Med J 1903;2(2239):1400.
3. Cotterill J. Stiffness of the great toe in adolescents. Br Med J 1887;1(1378):1158.
4. Hetherington VJ, Carnett J, Patterson BA. Motion of the first metatarsophalangeal joint. J Foot Surg 1989;28(1):13–9.
5. Sarrafian S. Functional anatomy of the foot and ankle. Anatomy of the Foot and Ankle 1993;375–425.
6. Hallinan J, Statum SM, Huang BK, et al. High-Resolution MRI of the First Metatarsophalangeal Joint: Gross Anatomy and Injury Characterization. Radiographics 2020;40(4):1107–24.

7. Lucas DE, Philbin T, Hatic S. The Plantar Plate of the First Metatarsophalangeal Joint:An Anatomical Study. Foot Ankle Spec 2014;7(2):108–12.

8. Sun T, Li Q, Wang L, et al. Ossification timeline of sesamoid bones at metatarsophalangeal joints. Anat Sci Int 2021;96(1):55–61.

9. Drago S, Nazaroff H, Britton J, et al. Assessment and Management of Atraumatic First Metatarsophalangeal Joint Pain. J Am Acad Orthop Surg 2023;31(14):708–16.

10. Waldrop NE 3rd, Zirker CA, Wijdicks CA, et al. Radiographic evaluation of plantar plate injury: an in vitro biomechanical study. Foot Ankle Int 2013;34(3):403–8.

11. Dedmond BT, Cory JW, McBryde A Jr. The hallucal sesamoid complex. J Am Acad Orthop Surg 2006;14(13):745–53.

12. Nery C, Baumfeld D, Umans H, et al. MR Imaging of the Plantar Plate: Normal Anatomy, Turf Toe, and Other Injuries. Magn Reson Imaging Clin N Am 2017;25(1):127–44.

13. Hamilton WG. Stenosing tenosynovitis of the flexor hallucis longus tendon and posterior impingement upon the os trigonum in ballet dancers. Foot Ankle 1982;3(2):74–80.

14. Kirane YM, Michelson JD, Sharkey NA. Contribution of the flexor hallucis longus to loading of the first metatarsal and first metatarsophalangeal joint. Foot Ankle Int 2008;29(4):367–77.

15. Çatal B, Keskinbora M, Keskinöz EN, et al. Is denervation surgery possible in the treatment of hallux rigidus? An anatomic study of cadaveric specimens. Acta Orthop Traumatol Turcica 2021;55(4):327–31.

16. UP Wyss, McBride I, Murphy L, et al. Joint reaction forces at the first MTP joint in a normal elderly population. J Biomech 1990;23(10):977–84.

17. Stokes IA, Hutton WC, Stott JR. Forces acting on the metatarsals during normal walking. J Anat 1979;129(Pt 3):579–90.

18. Jacob HA. Forces acting in the forefoot during normal gait–an estimate. Clin Biomech 2001;16(9):783–92.

19. Shereff MJ, Bejjani FJ, Kummer FJ. Kinematics of the first metatarsophalangeal joint. J Bone Joint Surg Am 1986;68(3):392–8.

20. Caravelli S, Mosca M, Massimi S, et al. A comprehensive and narrative review of historical aspects and management of low-grade hallux rigidus: conservative and surgical possibilities. Musculoskelet Surg 2018;102(3):201–11.

21. Sánchez-Gómez R, Becerro-de-Bengoa-Vallejo R, Losa-Iglesias ME, et al. Reliability Study of Diagnostic Tests for Functional Hallux Limitus. Foot Ankle Int 2020;41(4):457–62.

22. Bojsen-Møller F, Lamoreux L. Significance of free-dorsiflexion of the toes in walking. Acta Orthop Scand 1979;50(4):471–9.

23. Cody EA, Kraszewski AP, Marinescu A, et al. Measuring Joint Flexibility in Hallux Rigidus Using a Novel Flexibility Jig. Foot Ankle Int 2017;38(8):885–92.

24. Gajdosik RL, Bohannon RW. Clinical measurement of range of motion. Review of goniometry emphasizing reliability and validity. Phys Ther 1987;67(12):1867–72.

25. Michelson J, Dunn L. Tenosynovitis of the flexor hallucis longus: a clinical study of the spectrum of presentation and treatment. Foot Ankle Int 2005;26(4):291–303.

26. Vulcano E, Tracey JA 3rd, Myerson MS. Accurate Measurement of First Metatarsophalangeal Range of Motion in Patients With Hallux Rigidus. Foot Ankle Int 2016;37(5):537–41.

27. Betts R, Franks C, Duckworth T. Foot pressure studies: normal and pathological gait analysis. Disorders of the foot and ankle 1991;1:484–579.

28. Canseco K, Long J, Marks R, et al. Quantitative motion analysis in patients with hallux rigidus before and after cheilectomy. J Orthop Res 2009;27(1):128–34.
29. Canseco K, Long J, Marks R, et al. Quantitative characterization of gait kinematics in patients with hallux rigidus using the Milwaukee foot model. J Orthop Res : official publication of the Orthopaedic Research Society 2008;26(4):419–27.
30. Cansel AJM, Stevens J, Bijnens W, et al. Hallux rigidus affects lower limb kinematics assessed with the Gait Profile Score. Gait Posture 2021;84:273–9.
31. Colò G, Fusini F, Samaila EM, et al. The efficacy of shoe modifications and foot orthoses in treating patients with hallux rigidus: a comprehensive review of literature. Acta Biomed 2020;91(14-s):e2020016.
32. Colò G, Fusini F, Zoccola K, et al. May footwear be a predisposing factor for the development of hallux rigidus? A review of recent findings. Acta Biomed 2021; 92(S3):e2021010.
33. Lawrence JS, Bremner JM, Bier F. Osteo-arthrosis. Prevalence in the population and relationship between symptoms and x-ray changes. Ann Rheum Dis 1966; 25(1):1–24.
34. Roddy E, Thomas MJ, Marshall M, et al. The population prevalence of symptomatic radiographic foot osteoarthritis in community-dwelling older adults: cross-sectional findings from the clinical assessment study of the foot. Ann Rheum Dis 2015;74(1):156–63.
35. Bergin SM, Munteanu SE, Zammit GV, et al. Impact of first metatarsophalangeal joint osteoarthritis on health-related quality of life. Arthritis Care Res 2012;64(11): 1691–8.
36. Anderson MR, Ho BS, Baumhauer JF. Republication of "Current Concepts Review: Hallux Rigidus". Foot Ankle Orthop 2023;8(3). 24730114231188123.
37. Gould N, Schneider W, Ashikaga T. Epidemiological Survey of Foot Problems in the Continental United States: 1978–1979. Foot Ankle 1980;1(1):8–10.
38. Coughlin MJ, Shurnas PS. Hallux rigidus. Grading and long-term results of operative treatment. J Bone Joint Surg Am 2003;85(11):2072–88.
39. Howard N, Cowen C, Caplan M, et al. Radiological prevalence of degenerative arthritis of the first metatarsophalangeal joint. Foot Ankle Int 2014;35(12): 1277–81.
40. Wilder FV, Barrett JP, Farina EJ. The association of radiographic foot osteoarthritis and radiographic osteoarthritis at other sites. Osteoarthritis Cartilage 2005;13(3): 211–5.
41. van Saase JL, van Romunde LK, Cats A, et al. Epidemiology of osteoarthritis: Zoetermeer survey. Comparison of radiological osteoarthritis in a Dutch population with that in 10 other populations. Ann Rheum Dis 1989;48(4):271–80.
42. Coughlin MJ, Shurnas PS. Hallux rigidus: demographics, etiology, and radiographic assessment. Foot Ankle Int 2003;24(10):731–43 [published Online First: Epub Date]|.
43. Mann RA, Coughlin MJ, DuVries HL. Hallux rigidus: A review of the literature and a method of treatment. Clin Orthop Relat Res 1979;(142):57–63.
44. McMaster MJ. The pathogenesis of hallux rigidus. J Bone Joint Surg Br 1978; 60(1):82–7.
45. Horton GA, Park YW, Myerson MS. Role of metatarsus primus elevatus in the pathogenesis of hallux rigidus. Foot Ankle Int 1999;20(12):777–80.
46. Bonney G, Macnab I. Hallux valgus and hallux rigidus; a critical survey of operative results. J Bone Joint Surg Br 1952;34-b(3):366–85.
47. Jack EA. The aetiology of hallux rigidus. Br J Surg 1940;27(107):492–7.

48. Bingold AC, Collins DH. Hallux rigidus. J Bone Joint Surg Br 1950;32-b(2): 214–22.
49. Drago JJ, Oloff L, Jacobs AM. A comprehensive review of hallux limitus. J Foot Surg 1984;23(3):213–20.
50. Viegas GV. Reconstruction of hallux limitus deformity using a first metatarsal sagittal-Z osteotomy. J Foot Ankle Surg 1998;37(3):204–11, discussion 61-2.
51. Lundeen RO, Rose JM. Sliding oblique osteotomy for the treatment of hallux abducto valgus associated with functional hallux limitus. J Foot Ankle Surg 2000; 39(3):161–7.
52. Schweitzer ME, Maheshwari S, Shabshin N. Hallux valgus and hallux rigidus: MRI findings. Clin Imag 1999;23(6):397–402.
53. Hunt KJ, Anderson RB. Biplanar proximal phalanx closing wedge osteotomy for hallux rigidus. Foot Ankle Int 2012;33(12):1043–50.
54. Bejarano-Pineda L, Cody EA, Nunley JA 2nd. Prevalence of Hallux Rigidus in Patients With End-Stage Ankle Arthritis. J Foot Ankle Surg 2021;60(1):21–4 [published Online First: Epub Date]|.
55. Stein G, Pawel A, Koebke J, et al. Morphology of the first metatarsal head and hallux rigidus: a cadaveric study. Surg Radiol Anat 2012;34(7):589–92.
56. Goodfellow J. Aetiology of hallux rigidus. Proc Roy Soc Med 1966;59(9):821–4.
57. Nilsonne H. Hallux rigidus and its treatment. Acta Orthop Scand 1930;1(1–4): 295–303.
58. Calvo A, Viladot R, Giné J, et al. The importance of the length of the first metatarsal and the proximal phalanx of hallux in the etiopathogeny of the hallux rigidus. Foot Ankle Surg 2009;15(2):69–74.
59. Gerbert J, Moadab A, Rupley KF. Youngswick-Austin procedure: the effect of plantar arm orientation on metatarsal head displacement. J Foot Ankle Surg 2001;40(1):8–14.
60. Kilmartin TE. Phalangeal osteotomy versus first metatarsal decompression osteotomy for the surgical treatment of hallux rigidus: a prospective study of age-matched and condition-matched patients. J Foot Ankle Surg 2005;44(1):2–12.
61. Lambrinudi C. Metatarsus Primus Elevatus. Proc Roy Soc Med 1938;31(11):1273.
62. Meyer JO, Nishon LR, Weiss L, et al. Metatarsus primus elevatus and the etiology of hallux rigidus. J Foot Surg 1987;26(3):237–41.
63. Sanchez PJ, Grady JF, Lenz RC, et al. Metatarsus Primus Elevatus Resolution After First Metatarsophalangeal Joint Arthroplasty. J Am Podiatr Med Assoc 2018; 108(3):200–4.
64. Morton DJ. Hypermobility of the first metatarsal bone: the interlinking factor between metatarsalgia and longitudinal arch strains. JBJS 1928;10(2).
65. Klaue K, Hansen ST, Masquelet AC. Clinical, quantitative assessment of first tarsometatarsal mobility in the sagittal plane and its relation to hallux valgus deformity. Foot Ankle Int 1994;15(1):9–13.
66. Coughlin MJ, Shurnas PJ. Soft-tissue arthroplasty for hallux rigidus. Foot Ankle Int 2003;24(9):661–72.
67. Greisberg J, Sperber L, Prince DE. Mobility of the first ray in various foot disorders. Foot Ankle Int 2012;33(1):44–9.
68. Harris RI, Beath T. Hypermobile flat-foot with short tendo achillis. J Bone Joint Surg Am 1948;30a(1):116–40.
69. Bryant A, Tinley P, Singer K. A comparison of radiographic measurements in normal, hallux valgus, and hallux limitus feet. J Foot Ankle Surg 2000;39(1): 39–43.

70. Hintermann B, Nigg BM, Sommer C. Foot movement and tendon excursion: an in vitro study. Foot Ankle Int 1994;15(7):386–95.

71. Saggini R, Colotto S, Innocenti M. [Presence of a nucleus of distal ossification of the first metatarsus and its correlation with the pathogenesis of juvenile hallux rigidus]. Arch 'Putti' Chir Organi Mov 1984;34:59–69.

72. Pittman SR, Burns DE. The Wilson bunion procedure modified for improved clinical results. J Foot Surg 1984;23(4):314–20.

73. Youngswick FD. Modifications of the Austin bunionectomy for treatment of metatarsus primus elevatus associated with hallux limitus. J Foot Surg 1982;21(2):114–6.

74. Cavolo DJ, Cavallaro DC, Arrington LE. The Watermann osteotomy for hallux limitus. J Am Podiatry Assoc 1979;69(1):52–7.

75. Bouaicha S, Ehrmann C, Moor BK, et al. Radiographic analysis of metatarsus primus elevatus and hallux rigidus. Foot Ankle Int 2010;31(9):807–14.

76. Jones MT, Sanders AE, DaCunha RJ, et al. Assessment of Various Measurement Methods to Assess First Metatarsal Elevation in Hallux Rigidus. Foot Ankle Orthop 2019;4(3). 2473011419875686.

77. Seiberg M, Felson S, Colson JP, et al. 1994 William J. Stickel Silver Award. Closing base wedge versus Austin bunionectomies for metatarsus primus adductus. J Am Podiatr Med Assoc 1994;84(11):548–63.

78. Anwander H, Alkhatatba M, Lerch T, et al. Evaluation of Radiographic Features Including Metatarsus Primus Elevatus in Hallux Rigidus. J Foot Ankle Surg 2022;61(4):831–5.

79. Cheung ZB, Myerson MS, Tracey J, et al. Weightbearing CT Scan Assessment of Foot Alignment in Patients With Hallux Rigidus. Foot Ankle Int 2018;39(1):67–74.

80. Lee HY, Lalevee M, Mansur NSB, et al. Multiplanar instability of the first tarsometatarsal joint in hallux valgus and hallux rigidus patients: a case-control study. Int Orthop 2022;46(2):255–63.

81. Lee HY, Mansur NS, Lalevee M, et al. Does metatarsus primus elevatus really exist in hallux rigidus? A weightbearing CT case-control study. Arch Orthop Trauma Surg 2023;143(2):755–61.

82. Lucas DE, Hunt KJ. Hallux Rigidus: Relevant Anatomy and Pathophysiology. Foot Ankle Clin 2015;20(3):381–9.

83. Waldrop NE 3rd. Assessment and Treatment of Sports Injuries to the First Metatarsophalangeal Joint. Foot Ankle Clin 2021;26(1):1–12.

Classification and Radiology

Yu Min Suh, MD*, Joshua N. Tennant, MD

KEYWORDS

- Hallux rigidus • Classification • Radiology • Metatarsophalangeal joint • Imaging

KEY POINTS

- The article discusses the classification systems for hallux rigidus, including the Coughlin and Shurnas, Hattrup and Johnson, Regnauld, and Roukis classifications. These systems categorize the condition based on clinical and radiographic findings, helping clinicians assess the severity of joint degeneration and guide treatment decisions.
- Radiological imaging plays a crucial role in the evaluation of hallux rigidus. Standard radiography, including weight-bearing foot radiographs, provides valuable information about joint space narrowing and osteophyte formation. Advanced imaging techniques such as MRI and computed tomography offer detailed visualization of soft tissues, cartilage, and bone, aiding in the assessment of associated pathologies and surgical planning.
- Radiological evaluation, most often with plain film radiographs, is a critical aspect of the appropriate workup and diagnosis of hallux rigidus. Likewise, the understanding and recognition of classification systems for hallux rigidus allows clinicians to improve patient care, communication with colleagues, and research.

BACKGROUND

Hallux rigidus is a degenerative condition affecting the metatarsophalangeal joint of the big toe, resulting in pain, stiffness, and limited range of motion. Accurate classification and radiological assessment of hallux rigidus play a crucial role in its diagnosis and treatment planning. This article aims to provide an overview of the classification systems used to categorize hallux rigidus and the role of radiological imaging techniques in its evaluation. The information presented here will assist clinicians, radiologists, and researchers in effectively diagnosing and managing hallux rigidus.

DISCUSSION
Classification of Hallux Rigidus

Classification systems play a crucial role in categorizing and characterizing the spectrum of hallux rigidus, facilitating clinical decision making and treatment planning. There are more than 10 classification systems currently used in the staging of hallux

Department of Orthopaedics, University of North Carolina at Chapel Hill, 3144 Bioinformatics Bldg, CB# 7055, Chapel Hill, NC 27599, USA
* Corresponding author.
E-mail address: YuMin.Suh@unchealth.unc.edu

Foot Ankle Clin N Am 29 (2024) 389–404
https://doi.org/10.1016/j.fcl.2023.09.009
1083-7515/24/© 2023 Elsevier Inc. All rights reserved.

foot.theclinics.com

rigidus.[1] Several classification systems have been proposed to assess the severity and progression of this condition based on clinical and radiographic findings. These classification systems aim to provide a standardized framework for understanding the various stages and subtypes of hallux rigidus, allowing for better communication among health care professionals and facilitating research on treatment outcomes. By classifying hallux rigidus, clinicians can more accurately determine the appropriate management strategies tailored to each patient's specific needs. This section explores the key classification systems used in the assessment of hallux rigidus, delving into their components, strengths, limitations, and clinical implications. A comprehensive understanding of these classification systems is paramount in providing individualized care and optimizing treatment outcomes for patients with hallux rigidus.

Hattrup and Johnson classification

The Hattrup and Johnson classification system was first proposed in 1988, and it is the most commonly published classification system in the orthopedic literature. It classifies hallux rigidus based on radiographic findings and joint space narrowing.[2] Clinical characteristics are not accounted for in this classification system **(Table 1) (Fig 1)**.[3]

Coughlin and Shurnas classification

The Coughlin and Shurnas classification system is widely used to classify hallux rigidus based on clinical and radiographic findings, and it is considered to be the current gold standard classification method.[3,5] Coughlin and colleagues[6] categorized the condition into 4 stages, ranging from mild to severe, based on the extent of joint degeneration and the presence of osteophytes. Stage 0 represents a prearthritic condition with no radiographic changes, while stage 4 indicates severe joint degeneration with extensive osteophyte formation and joint space narrowing. Specifically, each of the stages is characterized by several features[7] **(Table 2)**.

Coughlin and Shurnas make several important distinctions in the description of their classification system. They intentionally avoid measurements that incorporate ill-defined theories, such as hallux elevatus or functional hallux limitus. Range of motion measurements in this system are defined by passive motion. As an important factor that differentiates Grade 3 and Grade 4, pain at midrange of motion is defined as pain throughout the arc of motion between maximum plantarflexion and maximum dorsiflexion. Any grade can include osteochondral defects and loose bodies. Ranges of motion between grades have intentional overlap, to allow the grader to choose the appropriate grade based on all three3 criteria of range of motion, radiograph findings, and clinical examination.

The key finding that Coughlin and Shurnas note from their study is that of differentiating between Grade 3 and Grade 4 for deciding to treat with cheilectomy versus fusion. Out of 110 patients treated, all nine patients with Grade 4 hallux rigidus who underwent cheilectomy had a failed outcome. In contrast, only 2 of 34 patients with

Table 1	
Hattrup and Johnson classification	
Grade	Radiographic Finding
1	Mild-to-moderate osteophyte formation but with good joint space preservation
2	Moderate osteophyte formation with joint space narrowing and subchondral sclerosis
3	Marked osteophyte formation and loss of the visible joint space, ± subchondral cyst formation

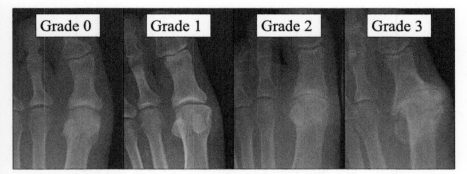

Fig. 1. Severity of hallux rigidus, graded according to Hattrup and Johnson classification system.[4].

Grade 3 hallux rigidus failed cheilectomy. The 2 failures of Grade 3 cheilectomies were found to be associated with less than 50% of metatarsal articular head cartilage remaining on intraoperative joint inspection.[8]

Regnauld classification

The Regnauld classification system[9] divides hallux rigidus into 3 grades based on radiographic findings. It focuses on joint space narrowing, osteophyte size, and subchondral sclerosis, providing a simplified yet informative approach to assessing disease severity.

> Grade I: mild limitation of dorsiflexion, mild dorsal spurring, pain, subchondral sclerosis (functional hallux limitus)
> Grade II: joint adaptation with flattening of the first metatarsal head and pain at the end range of motion, sesamoid hypertrophy
> Grade III: arthrosis with severe flattening of the first metatarsal head, osteophytes, asymmetric joint space narrowing, and erosions

Similarly to the Hattrup and Johnson classification systems, while this system delineates clear characteristics to look for radiologically regarding the first metatarsophalangeal joint, it fails to incorporate any clinical aspects of the disease.[3]

Roukis classification

Roukis classification is a valuable addition to the classification systems for hallux rigidus, proposed by Roukis in 2002.[10] Similar to the aforementioned systems, this system categorizes hallux rigidus into 4 stages based on radiographic findings[1]:

> Grade 1: metatarsus primus elevatus, periarticular subchondral sclerosis, minimal dorsal exostosis, and minimal flattening of the metatarsal head.
> Grade 2: moderate dorsal exostosis, flattening metatarsal head, minimal joint space narrowing, sesamoid hypertrophy
> Grade 3: severe dorsal exostosis, focal joint space narrowing, cyst formation, loose bodies
> Grade 4: excessive exostosis of the metatarsal head and proximal phalanx base, absent joint space, ankylosis

Radiological Evaluation of Hallux Rigidus

Radiological evaluation of hallux rigidus, like many orthopedic conditions, is central to understanding the nature and severity of the pathology. Plain film radiographs of the

Table 2
Adapted from Coughlin and Shurnas clinical radiographic system for grading hallux rigidus[7]

Grade	Dorsiflexion	Radiographic Findings	Clinical Findings
0	40° to 60° and/or 10% to 20% loss compared with normal side	Normal	No pain; only stiffness and loss of motion on examination
1	30° to 40° and/or 20% to 50% loss compared with normal side	Dorsal osteophyte is main finding, minimal joint space narrowing, minimal periarticular sclerosis, minimal flattening of metatarsal head	Mild or occasional pain and stiffness, pain at extremes of dorsiflexion and/or plantar flexion on examination
2	10° to 30° and/or 50% to 75% loss compared with normal side	Dorsal, lateral, and possibly medial osteophytes giving flattened appearance to metatarsal head, no more than $1/4$ if dorsal joint space involved on lateral radiograph, mild-to-moderate joint space narrowing and sclerosis, sesamoids not usually involved	Moderate-to-severe pain and stiffness that may be constant; pain occurs just before maximum dorsiflexion and maximum plantar flexion on examination
3	$\leq 10°$ and/or 75% to 100% loss compared with normal side. There is notable loss of metatarsophalangeal plantar flexion as well (often $\leq 10°$ of plantar flexion)	Same as in Grade 2 but with substantial narrowing, possibly periarticular cystic changes, more than $1/4$ of dorsal joint space involved on lateral radiograph, sesamoids enlarged and/or cystic and/or irregular	Nearly constant pain and substantial stiffness at extremes of range of motion but not at midrange
4	Same as in Grade 3	Same as in Grade 3; loose bodies and osteochondritis dessicans	Same criteria as Grade 3 but, there is definite pain at midrange of passive motion

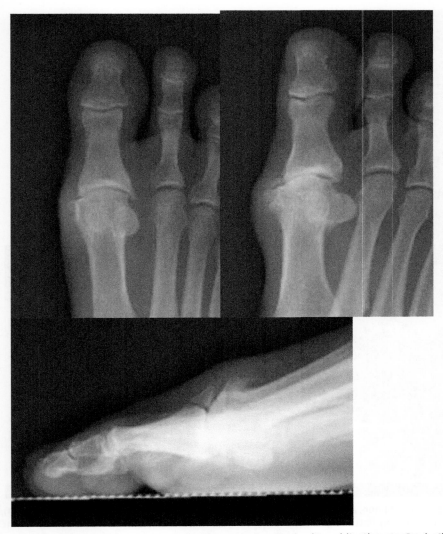

Fig. 2. AP, oblique, and lateral views of advanced hallux rigidus (Coughlin-Shurnas Grade 4), with narrowed joint space, dorsal metatarsal osteophyte, and dorsal loose body, which is potentially a fracture from the dorsal exostosis, at the dorsal joint.

foot have served as the imaging mainstay for the evaluation of hallux rigidus, and these remain a central foundation upon which the diagnosis and treatment plan are constructed. Advanced imaging techniques, such as MRI, computed tomography (CT), and ultrasonography also may play a role in imaging hallux rigidus.

Radiographs

Standard radiography, including weight-bearing anteroposterior (AP), lateral, and oblique views, is the initial imaging modality for evaluating hallux rigidus. It provides valuable information about joint space narrowing, joint incongruency, osteophyte formation, and the presence of other degenerative changes. Sesamoid views may be

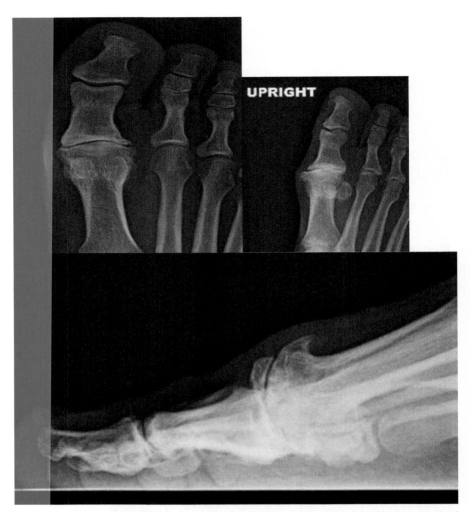

Fig. 3. AP, oblique, and lateral views of advanced hallux rigidus (Coughlin-Shurnas Grade 4), demonstrating flattening of the metatarsal head on the AP view, with enlargement of the dorsal metatarsal head.

used to assess sesamoid-metatarsal arthritis, including enlargement of the sesamoids, and alignment of the sesamoids on a standing sesamoid view. The AP and lateral weight-bearing views help assess joint alignment, while external oblique view is useful for identifying dorsomedial osteophytes.[11]

The typical radiograph findings are dorsal osteophyte formation on the head of the first metatarsal, narrowed joint space in the first MTP joint, flattened head of the first metatarsal, subchondral cysts and subchondral sclerosis.[12]

On the AP radiograph, arthritis and osteophyte formation are more typically visualized on the lateral rather than the medial aspect of the metatarsophalangeal joint. The lateral view of the foot may show a dorsal osteophyte that has the appearance of a breaking ocean wave flowing in the proximal direction along the dorsal metaphysis

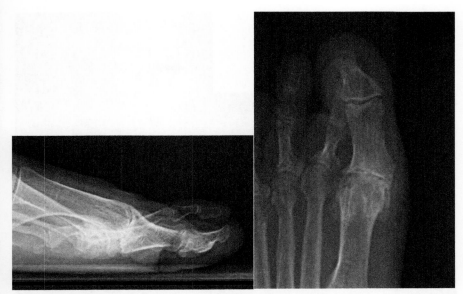

Fig. 4. 85-year-old woman with advanced hallux rigidus, demonstrating advancement of arthritis after cheilectomy 15 years earlier. Joint space is severely narrowed, but the dorsal osteophyte has been removed and has not regrown.

of the metatarsal. Fracture of the dorsal osteophyte may appear as a loose body at the dorsal joint. Overhang of the osteophyte on the AP view also may lead the viewer to believe that the joint is more narrowed and arthritic than it actually is. A dorsiflexion radiograph view may demonstrate dorsal bony impingement as the reason for limitation of great toe extension (**Figs. 2–8**).[13]

MRI
MRI is a noninvasive imaging technique that offers detailed visualization of soft tissues, cartilage, and bone marrow. It aids in the assessment of articular cartilage integrity, synovial inflammation, and ligamentous injuries associated with hallux rigidus. MRI is particularly useful in early-stage hallux rigidus, where subtle changes may not be evident on standard radiographs.

Munteanu and colleagues performed a cross-sectional study comparing the MRI images of 22 participants with first metatarsophalangeal joint osteoarthritis with healthy controls.[14] They found that hallux rigidus is associated with increased severity of osteophytes (dorsal and plantar metatarsal head, and dorsal proximal phalanx), bone marrow lesions (metatarsal head and proximal phalanx), cysts of the metatarsal head, effusion-synovitis (dorsal aspect), joint space narrowing (metatarsal-proximal phalanx and metatarsal-sesamoids), and cartilage loss. However, bone marrow lesions of the sesamoids, cysts of the proximal phalanx, and effusion-synovitis (plantar aspect) were found to be not significantly associated with metatarsophalangeal joint osteoarthritis (**Figs. 9 and 10**).

Magnetic resonance arthrography of the first metatarsophalangeal joint may also be considered for tertiary imaging evaluation (after radiographs and noncontrast MRI have not revealed a diagnosis) to increase sensitivity of the investigation. Enhanced visualization of intra-articular structures has been demonstrated with the addition of arthrography to MRI.[15] The painful first metatarsophalangeal joint with normal or

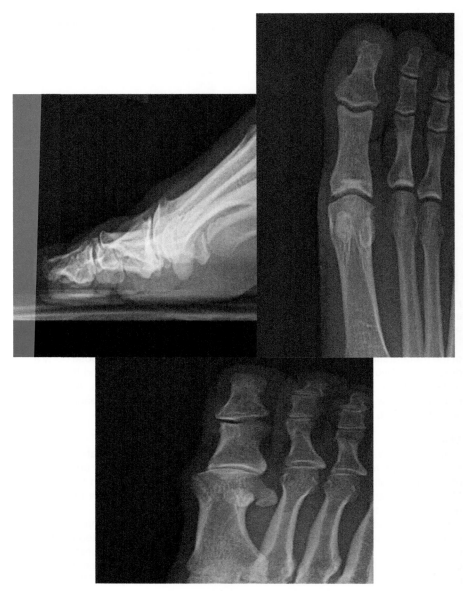

Fig. 5. AP, oblique, and lateral views of Coughlin-Shurnas Grade 1 hallux rigidus, demonstrating relatively preserved joint space with small dorsal osteophyte. Minimal osteophyte formation on medial and lateral aspects of the MTP joint.

minimally arthritic radiographs, with greater than expected symptoms, may have an unstable cartilage lesion or loose body that could be revealed with the use of contrast injected in the joint. A high index of suspicion for an intra-articular lesion that is not visible on other modalities, and expectation of patient tolerance of the arthrogram procedure, should be used to determine the limited indications for this imaging modality.

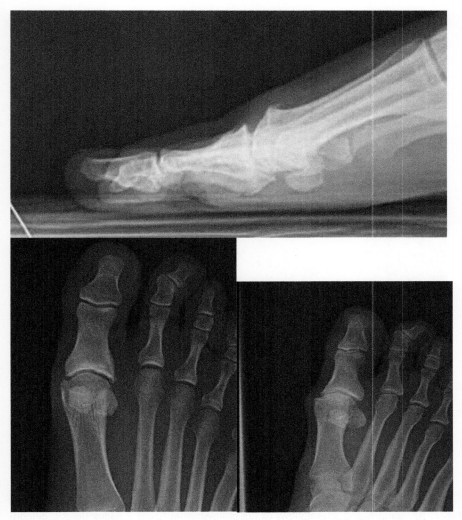

Fig. 6. AP, oblique, and lateral views of Coughlin-Shurnas Grade 2 hallux rigidus, demonstrating more narrowed joint space with dorsal, lateral, and medial osteophytes.

Computed tomography

CT scans provide cross-sectional images that can help evaluate the bony anatomy, osteophyte formation, and joint space narrowing in hallux rigidus. It is particularly useful in surgical planning for joint-sparing or joint-destructive procedures. CT scans, particularly those performed with the patient weight bearing, can also aid in identifying any associated deformities or joint malalignment.

Weight-bearing CT has been shown to specifically evaluate the presence of first metatarsal elevation, or metatarsus primus elevatus, in hallux rigidus. Lee and colleagues[16] found that those with symptomatic hallux rigidus were found to have significantly increased dorsal translation of the first metatarsal at the first tarsometatarsal joint. They established the diagnostic threshold as 4.19 mm on weight-bearing CT

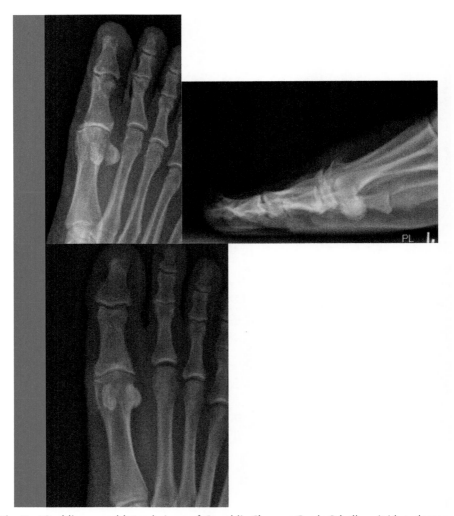

Fig. 7. AP, oblique, and lateral views of Coughlin-Shurnas Grade 3 hallux rigidus, demon-strating with significant joint space narrowing, flattening of the metatarsal head, cystic changes at the subchondral bone, and medial, lateral, and dorsal osteophytes.

with 77% sensitivity and 77% specificity. Cheung and colleagues found the degree of metatarsal elevation on weight-bearing CT to be greater in more severe cases of hallux rigidus (Coughlin and Shurnas grade 3 and 4 compared with 1 and 2).[17] By using 3-dimensional weight-bearing imaging, these studies were able to overcome the limitations of traditional 2-dimensional plain films in assessing metatarsal elevation caused by overlap of the metatarsals on the lateral view depending on the orientation of the foot and severity of the deformity (**Fig. 11**).

Finally, similar to plain films, CT images can be used in postoperative follow-up of first metatarsophalangeal fusion. There have been studies questioning the accuracy of plain films in successfully determining radiographic union after arthrodesis in the foot and ankle.[18] In cases where plain radiographs do not provide sufficient details

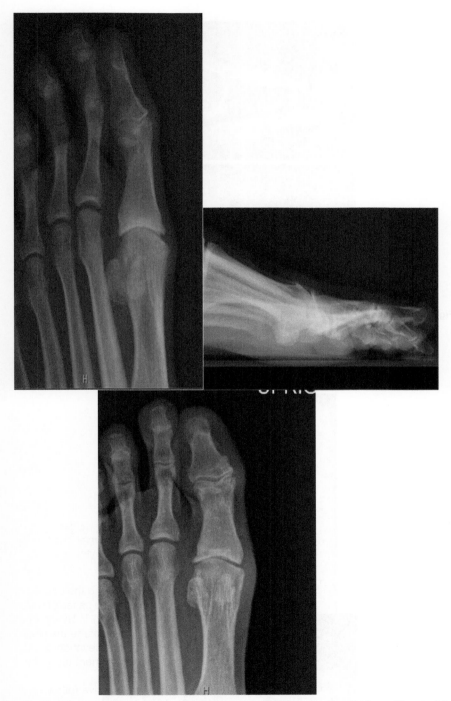

Fig. 8. AP, oblique, and lateral views of Coughlin-Shurnas Grade 3 hallux rigidus, with complete loss of joint space, most notable on the lateral view. Despite more significant narrowing, this remains Grade 3 rather than Grade 4, because the patient had a lack of pain at midrange of motion.

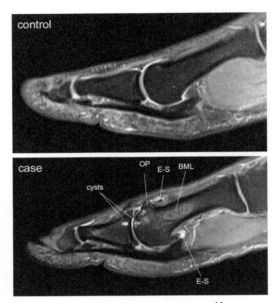

Fig. 9. MRI images of first MTP with arthritic characteristics.[14].

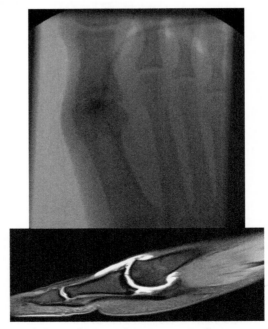

Fig. 10. First metatarsophalangeal joint arthrogram under fluoroscopy, followed by MRI to increase sensitivity in evaluating for loose bodies, unstable cartilage, and capsular injuries.

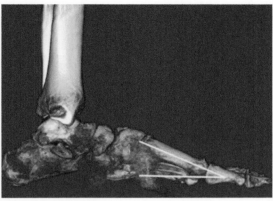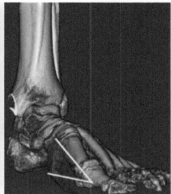

Fig. 11. 3-dimensional reconstruction of foot CT.[17].

to properly assess bony union, CT can be used to evaluate what percentage of the joint has been fused (**Fig. 12**).[19]

Ultrasonography

Ultrasonography is a dynamic imaging modality that can assess joint motion, synovial thickening, and the presence of soft tissue abnormalities. It is a cost-effective and readily available tool for diagnosing hallux rigidus. Ultrasonography can also be used to guide interventions such as joint injections or arthroscopic surgery in treating the first metatarsophalangeal joint. The first metatarsophalangeal joint is small to begin with, and the space is further narrowed by osteophytes and synovial scarring

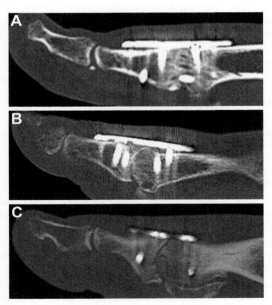

Fig. 12. Sagittal CT showing full fusion, partial fusion, and no fusion after first metatarsophalangeal arthrodesis.[19].

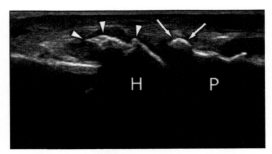

Fig. 13. Sonographic image of first metatarsophalangeal joint (H – first metatarsal head, P – proximal phalanx of the toe).[20]

in hallux rigidus. This can make it challenging for the provider to access the joint with a needle or a camera, affecting the efficacy of these interventions. Ultrasonographic guidance can aid minimally invasive procedures by allowing real-time visualization without the need for c-arm (**Fig. 13**).[20]

Moreover, ultrasound allows the visualization of not only bony but also soft tissue structures surrounding the first metatarsophalangeal joint, such as the capsular ligamentous sesamoid complex, plantar plate, flexor hallucis longus, and abductor and adductor hallucis tendons. The integrity of these structures may affect a provider's treatment decision.[21]

SUMMARY

Accurate classification and radiological assessment are essential in the diagnosis and management of hallux rigidus. Coughlin and Shurnas, Hattrup and Johnson, Regnauld, and Roukis classification systems provide valuable frameworks for categorizing hallux rigidus based on clinical and radiographic findings. Radiological imaging techniques, including standard radiography, MRI, CT, and ultrasonography, aid in evaluating the extent of joint degeneration, osteophyte formation, and associated soft tissue abnormalities. The information obtained through classification and radiological assessment guides treatment decisions in individuals with hallux rigidus.

CLINICS CARE POINTS

- The Coughlin and Shurnas classification system and Hattrup and Johnson, Regnauld, and Roukis classification systems, are useful tools for categorizing hallux rigidus based on radiographic findings. Understanding these classification systems can assist in determining the severity of joint degeneration and guiding treatment decisions.

- Radiographic evaluation, including weight-bearing AP, lateral, and oblique views, is crucial in the assessment of hallux rigidus. These views provide valuable information about joint space narrowing, osteophyte formation, and other degenerative changes.

- The anteroposterior weight-bearing view helps assess joint alignment, while the lateral view provides a clear visualization of the osteophytes and joint space narrowing. Oblique views can aid in identifying the presence and location of osteophytes.

- Radiographic findings can also help differentiate hallux rigidus from other conditions affecting the MTP joint, such as gout or rheumatoid arthritis. Careful evaluation of joint space narrowing, osteophyte formation, and the presence of joint erosion can provide valuable diagnostic clues.

- In cases where standard radiographs do not provide sufficient information, advanced imaging techniques such as MRI or CT may be considered. MRI offers detailed visualization of soft tissues, cartilage, and bone marrow, aiding in the assessment of associated ligamentous injuries or synovial inflammation. CT scans provide cross-sectional images that can help evaluate bony anatomy, osteophyte formation, and joint space narrowing, particularly for surgical planning purposes.
- Radiographic follow-up is essential in monitoring disease progression and treatment outcomes. Periodic imaging can help assess changes in joint space narrowing, osteophyte size, or the development of new joint deformities, guiding further management decisions.

DISCLOSURE

The authors have no commercial or financial conflicts of interest or any funding sources to declare.

REFERENCES

1. Dillard S, Schilero C, Chiang S, et al. Intra- and interobserver reliability of three classification systems for hallux rigidus. J Am Podiatr Med Assoc 2018. https://doi.org/10.7547/16-126.
2. Hattrup SJ, Johnson KA. Subjective results of hallux rigidus following treatment with cheilectomy. Clin Orthop Relat Res 1988;226:182–91.
3. Marcolli D. Hallux Rigidus: A Literature Review of Classifications, Etiology and Treatment. EC Orthopaedics 2019;10:874–91.
4. Senga Y, Nishimura A, Ito N, et al. Prevalence of and risk factors for hallux rigidus: a cross-sectional study in Japan. BMC Muscoskel Disord 2021;22:786.
5. Beeson P, Phillips C, Corr S, et al. Classification systems for hallux rigidus: a review of the literature. Foot Ankle Int 2008;29:407–14.
6. Coughlin MJ, Shurnas PS. Hallux rigidus: demographics, etiology, and radiographic assessment. Foot Ankle Int 2003;24(10):731–43. https://doi.org/10.1177/107110070302401002.
7. Lam A, Chan JJ, Surace MF, et al. Hallux rigidus: how do I approach it? World J Orthoped 2017;8(5):364–71.
8. Coughlin MJ, Shurnas PS. Hallux rigidus. Grading and long-term results of operative treatment. J Bone Joint Surg Am 2003;85(11):2072–88.
9. Regnauld B. The foot: pathology, aetiology, seminology, clinical investigation and therapy. New York: Springer-Verlag; 1986.
10. Roukis TS. Anatomic and biomechanical considerations in hallux rigidus. J Am Acad Orthop Surg 2022;10(5):347–57.
11. Bro NK, Lange J, Kabel JF. Ugeskr Laeger 2021;183(3):V08200627.
12. Smith RW, Katchis SD, Ayson LC, et al. Outcomes in hallux rigidus patients treated nonoperatively: a long-term follow-up study. Foot Ankle Int 2000;21(11):906–13.
13. Mann RA, Coughlin MJ, Salzmann C. Surgery of the foot and ankle. Philadelphia: Mosby Elsevier; 2007.
14. Munteanu SE, Auhl M, Tan JM, et al. Characterisation of first metatarsophalangeal joint osteoarthritis using magnetic resonance imaging. Clin Rheumatol 2021;40(12):5067–76.
15. Theumann NH, Pfirrmann CW, Mohana Borges AV, et al. Metatarsophalangeal joint of the great toe: normal MR, MR arthrographic, and MR bursographic findings in cadavers. J Comput Assist Tomogr 2002;26(5):829–38.

16. Lee HY, Mansur NS, Lalevee M, et al. Does metatarsus primus elevatus really exist in hallux rigidus? A weightbearing CT case-control study. Arch Orthop Trauma Surg 2023;143(2):755–61.
17. Cheung ZB, Myerson MS, Tracey J, et al. Weightbearing CT scan assessment of foot alignment in patients with hallux rigidus. Foot Ankle Int 2018;39(1):67–74.
18. Coughlin MJ, Grimes JS, Traughber PD, et al. Comparison of radiographs and CT scans in the prospective evaluation of the fusion of hindfoot arthrodesis. Foot Ankle Int 2006;27(10):780–7.
19. Wanivenhaus F, Espinosa N, Tscholl PM, et al. Quality of early union after first metatarsophalangeal joint arthrodesis. J Foot Ankle Surg 2017;56(1):50–3.
20. Paczesny ŁM, Kruczyński J. Ultrasound-guided arthroscopic management of hallux rigidus. Wideochir Inne Tech Maloinwazyjne 2016;11(3):144–8.
21. Chen X, Zhou G, Xue H, et al. High-resolution ultrasound of the forefoot and common pathologies. Diagnostics 2022;12(7):1541.

Hallux Rigidus
Update on Conservative Management

Antoine S. Acker, MD[a,b,*],
Kepler Alencar Mendes de Carvalho, MD[a],
Andrew E. Hanselman, MD[a]

KEYWORDS

• Hallux rigidus • Conservative • Orthotics • Injection • Therapy • Nonoperative

KEY POINTS

- The efficacy of conservative treatment for hallux rigidus is linked to initial pain levels.
- Although shoe modifications and insoles are common first-line treatments, their true effectiveness lacks strong evidence and physical therapy lack comprehensive guidance.
- Injection therapy, including corticosteroids and hyaluronic acid, exhibits varied outcomes, with about 50% of patients undergoing surgery within 1 to 2 years.
- The condition's etiology remains elusive, but recent biomechanical hypotheses hold promise.
- Understanding the disease's progression and exploring more effective conservative approaches is essential for optimal patient care.

INTRODUCTION

Hallux rigidus is a progressive degenerative arthritic condition affecting the first metatarsophalangeal (1st MTP) joint. Characterized by reduced joint mobility, pain, and the development of osteophytes, it presents a significant challenge for both patients and health care providers. Pain is likely a combination of cartilage loss, osteophyte formation/impingement, and joint inflammation. It is the second most common condition affecting the 1st MTP joint after hallux valgus and the most common form of arthritis in the foot. Women tend to be more affected than men, and bilateral presentation is common.

Before seeing a health care provider, most patients will have tried isolated oral therapy with nonsteroidal anti-inflammatories; however, it is usually insufficient for pain relief as the disease progresses. As it is often in orthopedics, this condition is initially

[a] Department of Orthopaedic Surgery, Research Scholar, Duke University, Durham, NC, USA;
[b] Centre of Foot and Ankle Surgery, Clinique La Colline, Geneva, Switzerland
* Corresponding author. Department of Orthopaedic Surgery, Duke University, 5601 Arringdon Park Dr, Morrisville, NC 27560-5643.
E-mail address: antoine.acker@duke.edu

Foot Ankle Clin N Am 29 (2024) 405–415
https://doi.org/10.1016/j.fcl.2023.09.010
1083-7515/24/© 2023 Elsevier Inc. All rights reserved.
foot.theclinics.com

treated with conservative measures and surgical treatment is considered when conservative measures fail to control the disease. There is a large array of surgical options from 1st MTP fusion to joint sparing procedures, such as osteotomies or joint replacement. It can be challenging to choose the right procedure for each patient, as most of them have important advantages and disadvantages, along with uncertainty for their short- and long-term outcomes. These surgical interventions will be covered in later sections throughout this review.

NOMENCLATURE

The condition was first described by Davies-Colley in 1887 as *hallux flexus*;[1] however, the current terminology of *hallux rigidus* was later described by Cotterill in 1903.[2] Although the term *rigidus* means "stiff" or "rigid" in Latin, most patients tend to seek medical treatment because of pain within the joint. From the perspective of the health care provider, a patient with a painful 1st MTP joint and some extent of degenerative changes will be diagnosed with hallux rigidus, regardless of the amount of motion.

Along with the term hallux rigidus, there are several other nomenclatures that need to be considered. Shariff and Myerson[3] introduced the concept of *functional hallux rigidus*, which is characterized by a reduced range of motion of the 1st MTP joint under weight-bearing or simulated weight-bearing conditions, but unrestricted motion of the 1st MTP joint in non-weight-bearing conditions. This is in contrast to *structural hallux rigidus*, which refers to restricted 1st MTP motion regardless of the weight-bearing condition. Another term to be familiar with is *hallux limitus*, which is often used but poorly defined. It may refer to a limitation of the 1st MTP motion without radiological signs of osteoarthritis,[4,5] but also tends to be used as a synonym of hallux rigidus.[6,7] Lam[8] suggested a better definition of *hallux limitus*, referring to it as "functional pain due to soft tissue tightness" without subsequent arthritic changes.

PREVALENCE

The prevalence of hallux rigidus has been reported from about 2.5% of the population older than 60 years in a 1980 epidemiologic survey from the United States[9] to 26.7% from a cohort study in Japan in 2021.[10] The discrepancy between these two studies may be explained as the 1980 survey was performed through patient questionnaires and the Japanese cohort study[10] assessed radiological and clinical findings. However, the overall ratio of symptomatic patients with radiological hallux rigidus in that particular cohort was 16.1%. This underlines the lack of correlation between the patient-reported outcomes/pain and the radiographic findings.[11] Another survey from the Netherlands,[12] as well as a more recent survey from the United States,[13] demonstrated a prevalence similar to that of the Japanese survey (**Table 1**).

LITERATURE UPDATE/LIMITATIONS

Hallux rigidus encompasses a large clinical spectrum, ranging from a mild degenerative joint in a young active patient to a highly degenerative stiff joint in an older and less active patient. Therefore, it is difficult to give precise recommendation for treatment. Less than 10% of the literature regarding hallux rigidus[14] discusses conservative treatment, and since the latest review in *Foot and Ankle clinics* in 2015,[15] no major contributions have been made.

Most studies referencing conservative treatments use clinical scores or conversion to surgery as an end point. While reviewing these studies, it is important to analyze how

Table 1
Prevalence of hallux rigidus in large epidemiological surveys

Author	Journal	Country	Total	Age (y) (SD)	Men	Women	Grade 1 (%)	Grade 2 (%)	Grade 3 (%)
Senga et al,[10] 2021	BMC MSK	Japan	604	67.1 (6.4)	208	110	19.0[a,b]	4.4[a,b]	2.1[a,b]
van Saase et al,[12] 1989	Ann of Rhe Dis	The Netherlands	312	50–54	312		Not reported	27.2	4.5
van Saase et al,[12] 1989	Ann of Rhe Dis	The Netherlands	85	70–74	85		Not reported	42.4	11.9
van Saase et al,[12] 1989	Ann of Rhe Dis	The Netherlands	298	50–54		298	Not reported	33.9	7
van Saase et al,[12] 1989	Ann of Rhe Dis	The Netherlands	122	70–74		122	Not reported	51.6	24.6
Wilder et al,[13] 2005	Osteo Cartil	USA	3436	62 (11)	25.1%	17.7%		20[c]	

a According to Hattrup and Johnson.[43]
b Symptomatic patients were, respectively, of 13.1%, 22.9 %, 14.2% for Grades 1–3.
c 2+ osteoarthritis.

many patients were ready to undergo surgical treatment. A study often quoted to support successful conservative treatment is a long-term longitudinal study by Smith.[16] Seventy-five percent of the patients would choose conservative treatment again, despite most of them not feeling improvement after treatment. Seventeen of 22 patients (77.7%) presented with a pain level not severe enough to proceed with surgical treatment. Also, studies with patient clinical scores as the end point seem to have the most restrictive inclusion criteria, such as relatively preserved range of motion or only mild to moderate degenerative changes. Last, there seems to be some confusion between hallux rigidus and hallux limitus within the literature. The term limitus may be used as a synonym for the term rigidus or it may be used to describe a painful 1st MTP joint with restricted motion but no arthritic degeneration, as stated earlier. This makes comparison of certain treatment modalities difficult within the literature.

ETIOLOGY

The etiology of hallux rigidus is poorly understood. Although there are many different theories, they are often conflicting with each other and lacking strong scientific evidence. Moving forward, a better understanding of the etiology is necessary and providers could optimize conservative treatment with the goal of slowing down the disease progression. Early on, anatomic or biomechanical abnormalities were suggested as possible etiologies: metatarsus primus elevatus,[17] long first metatarsal,[18] or pronation of the forefoot.[19] In the 1960s, Goodfellow[20] and McMaster proposed a post-traumatic etiology mainly based on observational case series with limited numbers and primarily young patients. Lately,[21,22] there has been a reemergence of a biomechanical etiology, specifically focusing on the structural and muscular imbalance leading to altered center of rotation of the 1st MTP joint. In 2008, a finite element analysis by Flavin[23] showed statistically significant evidence for an increase in tension of the plantar fascia resulting in cartilage damage on the articular surface. Maceira and Monteagudo[24] proposed a biomechanical hypothesis where the first metatarsophalangeal (1st MPT) joint motion occurred through a "gliding" motion instead of a "rolling" motion, secondary to a loss of the windlass mechanism and tightness of the Achilles–calcaneus–plantar system.

CLASSIFICATION

To date, no classification system of hallux rigidus has been regarded as a robust all-inclusive guide to predict treatment and outcomes.[25] Beeson and colleagues[25] identified 18 different classifications published since 1930 and most of them described only radiological findings. Roukis and colleagues[21] was the first system to include clinical and intraoperative features. Vanaore and colleagues[26] described a similar system with more emphasis on radiological criteria. Finally, Coughlin and Shurnas[27] built a classification system based on both radiological data as well as subjective and objective clinical examination with grades ranging from 0 to 4 (**Fig. 1**). A full discussion of the classifications is beyond the scope of this article and the readers are invited to read the review by Beeson and colleagues.[25] Future consideration may need to be given to the inclusion of both functional and structural hallux rigidus and the impact that these terms may have on joint-sparing and joint-sacrificing interventions.

EFFECTIVENESS OF CONSERVATIVE MANAGEMENT

How effective is conservative treatment of hallux rigidus in the long term? Again, research is limited. Smith and colleagues[16] published a longitudinal study based on

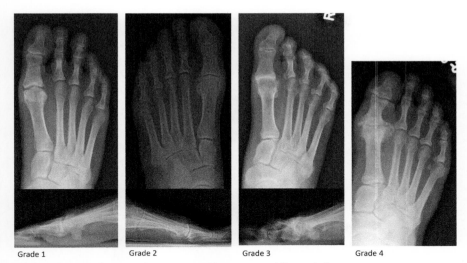

Grade 1   Grade 2   Grade 3   Grade 4

Fig. 1. Hallux rigidus classification according to Coughlin and Shurnas.

22 consecutive patients representing 24 feet with an average follow-up of 14.4 years (range 12–19 years). Seventy-three percent of the patients would choose a conservative treatment again, whereas 27% would have changed and chosen surgical treatment. Surgery was recommended in eight of those patients initially and 63% of them would make the same decision again. In regard to pain level, 92% of patients had no change in pain throughout the time period, with only one patient experiencing worsening pain and only one patient experiencing improvement of their pain, despite every joint showing some sort of cartilage loss with 33% having a loss of 2 mm or greater. In regard to treatment modalities, shoe modification with a larger/stiffer toe box was the most praised intervention. Three patients, however, reported that soft sole shoes were an effective measure. No injections were performed within this study group. Several reasons were given to explain the choice of choosing conservative treatment in this cohort, the most common reason being a tolerable pain level (77.7%) and many patients simply had objections in regard to the risks/consequences of surgical treatment.

INJECTION THERAPY

Manipulation under anesthesia was suggested by Watson Jones as a means to break down capsular adhesions.[28] This rarely used today in clinical practice. Corticosteroid injections tend to be more commonplace. Grice and colleagues reviewed 22 patients with hallux rigidus who received corticosteroid injection by a musculoskeletal radiologist under ultrasound or x-ray guidance. Twenty patients (91%) reported a benefit, but it was short-lived with only three patients (14%) reporting relief greater than 3 months. After 2 years, only two patients (9%) were asymptomatic, two patients (9%) had a second injection, and 12 patients (55%) required surgery. In a similar study, Solan[29] reported results on 37 patients with a minimum follow-up of 1 year after a corticosteroid injection (**Fig. 2**). Based on Karasick and Wapner's classification[30] (Grades 1–3), they found that patients with mild (Grade 1) and moderate (Grade 2) disease may benefit from intra-articular steroid injection with symptomatic pain relief at 6 weeks and 3 months, whereas patients with advanced disease (Grade 3) had little pain relief. Four of 12 patients with Grade 1

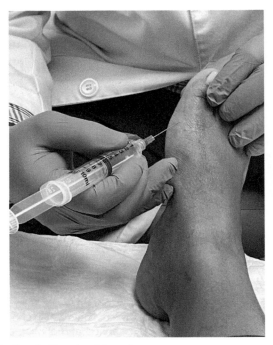

Fig. 2. 1st MTP injection (without guidance).

were scheduled for surgery, compared with 12 of 18 patients with Grade 2 disease, and five of five patients with Grade 3 disease. In general, corticosteroid injection for hallux rigidus seems to be less effective than other foot injection sites (ie, midfoot or hindfoot) and an improvement longer than 3 months can only be expected in patients with mild disease (Grade 1).

Hyaluronic acid (HA) has been tested as an alternative injection choice with little evidence supporting its effectiveness compared with corticosteroid in the long-term. A randomized trial compared HA (sodium hyaluronate) against corticosteroid (triamcinolone acetonide) in 37 patients with low-grade hallux rigidus.[31] At short-term follow-up (84 days), HA showed improved results compared with corticosteroid. At long-term follow-up (1 year), there was no difference between the groups. A larger randomized study,[32] with 151 patients and no inclusion limitation with regard to disease grading, demonstrated no advantage between HA (Hylan G-F 20) versus a placebo. In another study, repeated injection of 0.1 mL of acid hyaluronic on a weekly basis for 8 weeks showed reduction in pain level and improved range of motion in a population of golfers with a mean age of 70.5 years with any grade of hallux rigidus.[33] Subjective satisfaction and number of golf session per week also improved. Complications of MTP injection were reported as low and no patient-reported skin change and atrophy, but these complications were not specifically assessed in the follow-up questionnaire. Most patients who received an injection (see **Fig. 1**) were in their fifth decade of life. We chose not to add in-depth details regarding the changes in pain levels reported in these studies, given that the follow-up period ranged from 6 weeks to 1 year. Although patients experienced a change in pain, such a short follow-up period is not relevant for patients who likely expect to maintain an active lifestyle for at least 20 years. The conversion rate to surgery averaged around 50% after 1 or 2 years (**Table 2**).

Table 2
Conversion rate to surgery after the first metatarsophalangeal injection

Author	Journal	Product	(Follow-up (months)	Age (y) (SD or range)	Feet (n)	Grade 1 (n)[a]	Grade 2 (n)[a]	Grade 3 (n)[a]	Conversion to Surgery (%)
Solan et al,[29] 2001	JBJS Br	Corticosteroid	41.2	52.3 (11.04)	35	12	18	5	60[c]
Grice 2017	FAI	Corticosteroid	24	41 (14–82)[b]	22	Missing	Missing	Missing	54.5
Grady et al,[7] 2002	J Am Podiatr Med Assoc	Corticosteroid	>24	46 (17–78)	772	Missing	Missing	Missing	45
Pons et al,[31] 2007	FAI	Sodium hyaluronate	12	53.7 (11.3)	15	15	0	0	46.7
Pons et al,[31] 2007	FAI	Corticosteroid	12	55.3 (11.2)	17	17	0	0	52.9

[a] According to Karasick and Wapner.[28]
[b] Age range for the whole cohort of patients undergoing foot/ankle injection.
[c] Conversions rate were, respectively, 33.3%, 66.7%, and 100% for Grades 1–3.

PHYSICAL THERAPY

Physical therapy is a common first line of treatment in orthopedics. There is limited evidence about the effectiveness of physical therapy for hallux rigidus and the specific protocol that should be followed. In a Cochrane review in 2010,[34] only one published study was eligible as a trial. Shamus[5] reported pain reduction and improvement in function with sesamoid mobilization, flexor hallucis strengthening, gait training, and comprehensive physical therapy (calf and hamstring stretching, ultrasound, cold pack) compared with comprehensive therapy alone in 20 young patients (21–43 year old) with hallux limitus. There were several limitations with the study, specifically patients with bony proliferation were excluded from the study, they all had an acute trauma less than 1 year before the study, and the follow-up was only 4 weeks. These results are not generalizable to an older population with degenerative changes. In another study involving a large survey among physical therapists and podiatrists in Australia and the United Kingdom,[35] there were no specific treatment strategies for hallux rigidus and the treatments used were based on the evidence of osteoarthritis from other joints. The strategies from the physical therapist were massage, gait training, taping, joint manipulation, electrotherapy, acupuncture, and counseling on weight loss. None of these interventions have been studied and published for advanced stage of hallux rigidus.

Surprisingly no studies or recommendations exist on strengthening the peroneus longus, which flexes the first metatarsal. The personal experience of the one of our authors demonstrates a reduction on mild 1st MTP pain after daily strengthening the peroneus longus. Metatarsus primus elevatus is associated with hallux rigidus, and there are still controversies whether it is a causative factor[36] or a consequence of the degenerative changes. The flexor hallucis longus (FHL) is obviously involved in 1st MPT function and dysfunction.[37] It is unclear if the FHL tendon should be strengthened, as suggested by Shamus[5] or stretched.[38] There is also a lack of evidence regarding the mobilization of the MPT1 joint. Most studies[5,35] seek to improve the 1st MTP motion, but the patients studied tended to have low or mild degenerative changes.

SHOE MODIFICATION AND ORTHOTICS

High heels and tight shoes should be avoided as part of first-line treatment.[39] The most common shoe modification is a stiff rocker bottom sole and a large toe box, which are meant to decrease the 1st MTP motion during gait and to reduce irritation due to the osteophytes. Among patients that underwent conservative treatment for more than a decade, widened toe box was the most often praised shoe modification (13/22 patients), followed by avoidance of high heels (9/13 female patients). Stiffer soled shoes were praised by only five patients and soft sole shoes by three patients. Orthotics are also used to either limit the dorsiflexion of the 1st MTP joint motion through a Morton's extension[40] or plantarflex the first ray.[41] A randomized trial compared orthotics to rocker bottom shoes among 102 patients with a mean age of 57 years and degenerative changes on radiographs. Both groups showed, at 12 weeks follow-up, a similar reduction of pain level during walking and at rest. About 70% of the patients developed new back or lower extremity pain during the trial. Adherence to the treatment method was slightly higher in the orthotic group. A recent randomized trial[42] did not show any superiority between contoured foot orthoses versus sham insole in 88 patients with a mean age 61 year old. The two groups demonstrated a similar pain reduction after 12 weeks.

SUMMARY

There is a place for initial conservative treatment in most patients with hallux rigidus, understanding that there are limitations. These treatment options should be recommended in a tailored fashion based on patients' expectations and clinical and radiological findings. There is clearly a consensus that no conservative treatment can limit the degenerative evolution of the disease. Patients with a tolerable pain level may find a stabilization of their pain with conservative measures, despite worsening of their radiographic findings. For patients with high-grade degenerative changes and severe symptoms, there is no evidence to support a long lasting and efficient pain level reduction with injections, shoes modifications, or orthotics. These measures may stabilize the pain level over time but are unlikely to provide significant improvement. For patients with mild or moderate pain and degenerative changes, corticosteroid injections and shoe modification may provide pain relief for 3 to 6 months with long-lasting effect (>1 year) in only a limited number of patients. There is little evidence to support HA over corticosteroid in most patients; however, patients with mild degenerative changes, who are willing to have repeated injections on a short period of time, may benefit from HA as an alternative. There is no clear evidence to support physical therapy, and there is no specific protocol to follow. Most of the physical therapy protocols are based on the experience and habits of the physical theraptist.[35] There is a clearly a need for a better understanding of the etiology of the disease, to propose more efficient conservative treatment for patients who are either not eligible for surgery or reluctant to undergo a surgical treatment. This would also help to slow down the evolution of this degenerative condition.

CLINICS CARE POINTS

- Conservative treatment should always be considered when dealing with orthopedic pathology; however, providers should understand that the efficacy of conservative treatment for hallux rigidus is linked to initial pain levels.
- Although shoe modifications and insoles are common first-line treatments, their true effectiveness lacks strong evidence.
- Injection therapy demonstrates varied outcomes, with about 50% of patients undergoing surgery within 1 to 2 years.
- The condition's etiology remains elusive, but recent biomechanical hypotheses hold promise.
- Classifications and physical therapy lack comprehensive guidance.
- Understanding the disease's progression and exploring more effective conservative approaches is essential for optimal patient care.

DISCLOSURE

The authors have no commercial or financial conflicts of interest related to this work. All pictures and x-rays are from Dr Hanselman's records.

REFERENCES

1. Davies-Colley:Contraction of the metatarso-phalangealjoint of the great toe. Br Med J 1:728, 1887
2. Cotterill JM. The pathology of hallux rigidus. Br Med J 1903;2(2239):1400.

3. Shariff R, Myerson MS. The use of osteotomy in the management of Hallux Rigidus. Foot Ankle Clin 2015;20(3):493–502.

4. Lafuente G, Munuera PV, Dominguez G, et al. Hallux limitus and its relationship with the internal rotational pattern of the lower limb. J Am Podiatr Med Assoc 2011;101(6):467–74.

5. Shamus J, Shamus E, Gugel RN, et al. The effect of sesamoid mobilization, flexor hallucis strengthening, and gait training on reducing pain and restoring function in individuals with hallux limitus: a clinical trial. J Orthop Sports Phys Ther 2004; 34(7):368–76.

6. Shields J, Gambhir N, Alben M, et al. Cheilectomy with decompression osteotomy for treatment of hallux limitus and rigidus: a retrospective study with 5-year outcomes. J Foot Ankle Surg 2023;62(2):282–5.

7. Grady JF, Axe TM, Zager EJ, et al. A retrospective analysis of 772 patients with hallux limitus. J Am Podiatr Med Assoc 2002;92(2):102–8.

8. Lam A, Chan JJ, Surace MF, et al. Hallux rigidus: How do I approach it? World J Orthoped 2017;8(5):364–71.

9. Gould N, Schneider W, Ashikaga T. Epidemiological survey of foot problems in the continental United States: 1978-1979. Foot Ankle 1980;1(1):8–10.

10. Senga Y, Nishimura A, Ito N, et al. Prevalence of and risk factors for hallux rigidus: a cross-sectional study in Japan. BMC Muscoskel Disord 2021;22(1):786.

11. Nixon DC, Lorbeer KF, McCormick JJ, et al. Hallux rigidus grade does not correlate with foot and ankle ability measure score. J Am Acad Orthop Surg 2017; 25(9):648–53.

12. van Saase JL, van Romunde LK, Cats A, et al. Epidemiology of osteoarthritis: Zoetermeer survey. Comparison of radiological osteoarthritis in a Dutch population with that in 10 other populations. Ann Rheum Dis 1989;48(4):271–80.

13. Wilder FV, Barrett JP, Farina EJ. The association of radiographic foot osteoarthritis and radiographic osteoarthritis at other sites. Osteoarthritis Cartilage 2005;13(3):211–5.

14. Kon Kam King C, Loh Sy J, Zheng Q, et al. Comprehensive review of non-operative management of hallux rigidus. Cureus 20 2017;9(1):e987.

15. Kunnasegaran R, Thevendran G. Hallux rigidus: nonoperative treatment and orthotics. Foot Ankle Clin 2015;20(3):401–12.

16. Smith RW, Katchis SD, Ayson LC. Outcomes in hallux rigidus patients treated nonoperatively: a long-term follow-up study. Foot Ankle Int 2000;21(11):906–13.

17. Lambrinudi C. Metatarsus primus elevatus. Proc Roy Soc Med 1938;31(11):1273.

18. McMurray TP. Treatment of hallux valgus and rigidus. Br Med J 1936;2(3943):218–21.

19. Jansen M. Hallux valgus, rigidus, and malleus. J Orthop Surg 1921;3(3):87–90.

20. Goodfellow J. Aetiology of hallux rigidus. Proc Roy Soc Med 1966;59(9):821–4.

21. Roukis TS, Jacobs PM, Dawson DM, et al. A prospective comparison of clinical, radiographic, and intraoperative features of hallux rigidus: short-term follow-up and analysis. J Foot Ankle Surg 2002;41(3):158–65.

22. Dananberg HJ. Functional hallux limitus and its relationship to gait efficiency. J Am Podiatr Med Assoc 1986;76(11):648–52.

23. Flavin R, Halpin T, O'Sullivan R, et al. A finite-element analysis study of the metatarsophalangeal joint of the hallux rigidus. J Bone Joint Surg Br 2008;90(10):1334–40.

24. Maceira E, Monteagudo M. Functional hallux rigidus and the Achilles-calcaneus-plantar system. Foot Ankle Clin 2014;19(4):669–99.

25. Beeson P, Phillips C, Corr S, et al. Classification systems for hallux rigidus: a review of the literature. Foot Ankle Int 2008;29(4):407–14.
26. Vanore JV, Christensen JC, Kravitz SR, et al. Diagnosis and treatment of first metatarsophalangeal joint disorders. Section 2: Hallux rigidus. J Foot Ankle Surg 2003;42(3):124–36.
27. Coughlin MJ, Shurnas PS. Hallux rigidus. Grading and long-term results of operative treatment. J Bone Joint Surg Am 2003;85(11):2072–88.
28. Miettinen Mikko, Ramo Lasse, Lahdeoja Tuomas. Treatment of hallux rigidus (letter). BMJ 1927;1:1165–6.
29. Solan MC, Calder JD, Bendall SP. Manipulation and injection for hallux rigidus. Is it worthwhile? J Bone Joint Surg Br 2001;83(5):706–8.
30. Karasick D, Wapner KL. Hallux rigidus deformity: radiologic assessment. AJR Am J Roentgenol 1991;157(5):1029–33.
31. Pons M, Alvarez F, Solana J, et al. Sodium hyaluronate in the treatment of hallux rigidus. A single-blind, randomized study. Foot Ankle Int 2007;28(1):38–42.
32. Munteanu SE, Zammit GV, Menz HB, et al. Effectiveness of intra-articular hyaluronan (Synvisc, hylan G-F 20) for the treatment of first metatarsophalangeal joint osteoarthritis: a randomised placebo-controlled trial. Ann Rheum Dis 2011; 70(10):1838–41.
33. Petrella RJ, Cogliano A. Intra-articular hyaluronic acid treatment for Golfer's Toe: keeping older golfers on course. Phys Sportsmed 2004;32(7):41–5.
34. Zammit GV, Menz HB, Munteanu SE, et al. Interventions for treating osteoarthritis of the big toe joint. Cochrane Database Syst Rev 2010;(9):CD007809.
35. Paterson KL, Hinman RS, Menz HB, et al. Management of first metatarsophalangeal joint osteoarthritis by physical therapists and podiatrists in Australia and the United Kingdom: a cross-sectional survey of current clinical practice. J Foot Ankle Res 2020;13(1):14.
36. Bouaicha S, Ehrmann C, Moor BK, et al. Radiographic analysis of metatarsus primus elevatus and hallux rigidus. Foot Ankle Int 2010;31(9):807–14.
37. Kirane YM, Michelson JD, Sharkey NA. Contribution of the flexor hallucis longus to loading of the first metatarsal and first metatarsophalangeal joint. Foot Ankle Int 2008;29(4):367–77.
38. Michelson JD, Bernknopf JW, Charlson MD, et al. What is the efficacy of a nonoperative program including a specific stretching protocol for flexor hallucis longus tendonitis? Clin Orthop Relat Res 2021;479(12):2667–76.
39. Elattar O, Smith T, Ferguson A, et al. Republication of "uses of braces and orthotics for conservative management of foot and ankle disorders". Foot Ankle Orthop 2023;8(3). 24730114231193419.
40. Sammarco VJ, Nichols R. Orthotic management for disorders of the hallux. Foot Ankle Clin 2005;10(1):191–209.
41. Scherer PR, Sanders J, Eldredge DE, et al. Effect of functional foot orthoses on first metatarsophalangeal joint dorsiflexion in stance and gait. J Am Podiatr Med Assoc 2006;96(6):474–81.
42. Paterson KL, Hinman RS, Metcalf BR, et al. Effect of foot orthoses vs sham insoles on first metatarsophalangeal joint osteoarthritis symptoms: a randomized controlled trial. Osteoarthritis Cartilage 2022;30(7):956–64.
43. Hattrup SJ, Johnson KA. Subjective results of hallux rigidus following treatment with cheilectomy. Clin Orthop Relat Res 1988;226:182–91.

Dorsal Cheilectomy

Aaron T. Scott, MD

KEYWORDS

- Hallux rigidus • Dorsal cheilectomy • Metatarsophalangeal joint • Arthritis

KEY POINTS

- Resect the dorsal osteophyte, along with 25% to 30% of the first metatarsal head. Avoid resecting more than this amount to decrease the chances of developing instability.
- Resect kissing osteophyte off of the dorsal base of the proximal phalanx.
- Strive to achieve at least 50° of passive dorsiflexion through the first metatarsophalangeal joint after cheilectomy. Consider addition of a Moberg osteotomy in cases where this level of dorsiflexion is not achieved.
- Early patient-directed dorsiflexion and plantarflexion range of motion is essential to achieving a satisfactory result.

INTRODUCTION

The term "cheilectomy" is derived from the Greek word "cheilos" meaning "lip," and refers to a surgical resection of the dorsal osteophyte from the first metatarsal head. It is most often performed in patients with hallux rigidus,[1–3] who have less to no midrange pain of the first metatarsophalangeal (MTP) joint and who have failed nonoperative management.[4,5] Cheilectomy has been recommended for Shurnas and Coughlin Grades 1 and 2, as well as, Grade 3 hallux rigidus when greater than 50% of the articular surface of the first metatarsal head displays intact cartilage.[4] The procedure is simple, quick, and allows for maintained range of motion and strength.[5–7] Additional proposed advantages of the dorsal cheilectomy include low morbidity,[2,6,7] quicker postoperative recovery,[6] avoidance of costly implants, and the fact that the procedure does not inhibit future conversion to an arthrodesis.[5] These proposed advantages have led some authors to advocate for the use of a cheilectomy, even in patients with more extensive disease.[4,6] Although the technique described in the current article involves a standard dorsal incision, other authors have advocated for medial approaches[8] and minimally invasive techniques.[9]

PREOPERATIVE ASSESSMENT

Preoperatively, patients are assessed for the chronicity and severity of their symptoms. Earlier treatments, such as oral or topical medications, orthotics, carbon fiber

Department of Orthopaedic Surgery, Wake Forest University School of Medicine, Watlington Hall, 4th Floor, 1 Medical Center Boulevard, Winston-Salem, NC 27157, USA
E-mail address: aascott@wakehealth.edu

Foot Ankle Clin N Am 29 (2024) 417–424
https://doi.org/10.1016/j.fcl.2023.10.003
1083-7515/24/© 2023 Elsevier Inc. All rights reserved.

inserts, and injections are reviewed, and a thorough assessment of medical comorbidities is performed. Diabetes should be well controlled and smoking cessation should be emphasized, as necessary. In patients with inflammatory arthropathies, connective tissue disorders, and neuromuscular conditions, strong consideration should be given to a first MTP arthrodesis, if there is any associated deformity present.

Physical examination primarily focuses on an assessment of first MTP joint range of motion. The presence of end-range pain, in either full dorsiflexion or full plantarflexion, is noted. The presence of midrange pain warrants consideration of a first MTP arthrodesis.

Plain radiographs typically suffice. On anterior-posterior (AP) images (**Fig. 1**), assess alignment and joint space narrowing, as well as, the presence and size of subchondral cysts. Lateral images (**Fig. 2**) are used to assess for the presence and size of osteophytes emanating off of the first metatarsal head and base of the proximal phalanx. Moreover, oblique images may offer additional information regarding the presence of fibular metatarso-sesamoid arthrosis.

SURGICAL TECHNIQUE

Although general anesthesia may be used, regional anesthesia and sedation is preferable. The patient is placed in a supine position, and either a standard thigh tourniquet

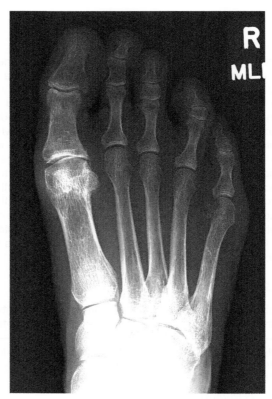

Fig. 1. Standard anteroposterior weight-bearing radiograph demonstrating joint-space narrowing and marginal osteophyte formation.

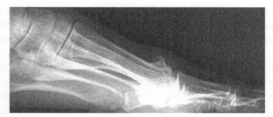

Fig. 2. Lateral weight-bearing radiograph demonstrating first metatarsal dorsal osteophyte formation, along with a loose body and marginal osteophyte emanating off of the base of the proximal phalanx.

or ankle Esmarch tourniquet may be used. However, if an ankle tourniquet is used, this should be removed before an assessment of first MTP joint range of motion following completion of the cheilectomy.

A dorsal longitudinal incision is centered on the first metatarsal head (**Fig. 3**) and is carried down to the level of the joint capsule. The capsule is incised in-line with the skin incision 5 mm medial to the extensor hallucis longus (EHL) tendon. Creating the arthrotomy well medial to the EHL tendon avoids damage to the tendon, reduces the formation of adhesions to the tendon, and allows for adequate capsular tissue

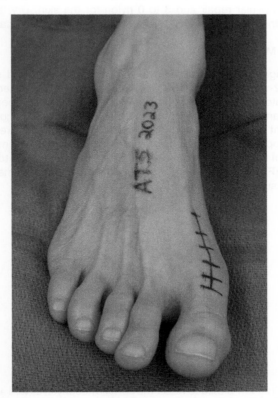

Fig. 3. Dorsal longitudinal incision centered on the first metatarsal head.

for final closure at the end of the procedure. The capsule is carefully elevated dorsally to expose the distal first metatarsal and the base of the proximal phalanx. Inflamed, hypertrophic synovial tissue is resected and any associated loose bodies are removed at this time.

The hallux is plantarflexed and the extent of articular cartilage damage is assessed. A fine-kerf sagittal saw is used to obliquely resect the dorsal osteophyte, as well as, the dorsal 25% to 33% of the first metatarsal head (**Fig. 4**). This amount of resection will often remove a portion of the full-thickness cartilage loss of the head and allows for increased dorsiflexion motion. The edges of the resection site may be smoothed with the saw, a small rongeur, or a small rasp. Small, well-contained first metatarsal (MT) head osteochondral defects may be "microfractured" with a 1.6 mm K-wire. A small amount of bone wax may be applied to the exposed cancellous surface to reduce early postoperative bleeding (**Fig. 5**). The joint is irrigated to remove small loose spicules of bone and excess wax. If a "kissing" dorsal osteophyte is present at the base of the proximal phalanx, this is removed with a small rongeur flush with the native dorsal rim of the phalangeal base (**Fig. 6**). Additionally, marginal osteophytes are removed medially and laterally with the rongeur or small hand osteotome.

The ankle tourniquet (if used) is removed at this juncture and range of motion of the first MTP joint is assessed (**Fig. 7**). If less than 50° of passive dorsiflexion is achieved, consideration should be given to a dorsal closing wedge osteotomy[10,11] (Moberg or Kessel-Bonney Osteotomy) of the proximal phalanx.

Final hemostasis is secured and the wound is closed in layered fashion using 2 to 0 vicryl for the capsular repair and 3 to 0 nylon for the skin. Dry, sterile dressings are applied and the patient is placed into a well-padded short leg cast.

POSTOPERATIVE MANAGEMENT

Limited heel weight-bearing is allowed in the cast. The cast and sutures may be removed at the 2-week postoperative visit, and the patient may then be placed into a hard-soled postop shoe. At this point, patients are instructed to begin gentle dorsiflexion and plantarflexion range of motion exercises of the first MTP joint, and they are allowed to weight bear as tolerated. Postoperative radiographs are not necessary. However, if postoperative radiographs are obtained, they should demonstrate appropriate resection of the dorsal osteophyte, along with the dorsal 25% to 33% of the first metatarsal head (**Fig. 8**). Moreover, most patients may return to normal shoewear by 4 to 6 weeks after surgery.

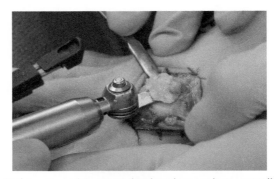

Fig. 4. A small sagittal saw is used to resect the dorsal osteophyte, as well as, the dorsal 25% to 30% of the first metatarsal head.

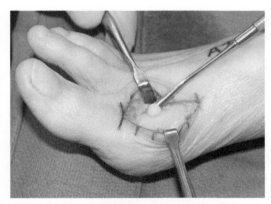

Fig. 5. Bone wax is applied to the cancellous bone at the resection site.

COMPLICATIONS

- Cellulitis[4,6,8]
- Progression of disease/recurrence[1,4,7]
- Stiffness[1]
- Persistent pain and need for subsequent arthrodesis[5,6]
- Deep venous thrombosis[12]
- Painful scar formation[12]
- Nerve injury/neuroma formation[7,8,12]
- Complex regional pain syndrome[7,12]

RESULTS

In 1930, Nilsonne reported on 2 patients that underwent dorsal cheilectomy for hallux rigidus, and thought that the procedure did "not leave a permanent result."[3] Therefore, and without any outcomes provided, the author "discarded these palliative methods," and instead opted, in the future, for resection arthroplasty. Retrospective reviews by Blair[13] and Durrant[14] also supported this view that the results of cheilectomy were only temporary. Moreover, Bonney and McNab reported poor results as well, stating that the results of the excision of the bony exostosis were "as poor as those of

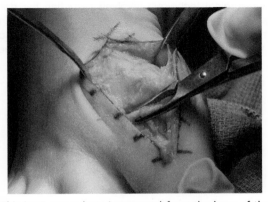

Fig. 6. The dorsal "kissing" osteophyte is removed from the base of the proximal phalanx with a small rongeur.

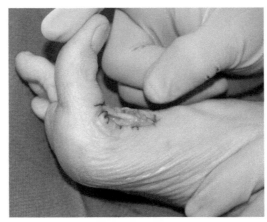

Fig. 7. Following the cheilectomy, the ankle tourniquet is removed and range of motion is assessed. The goal is to attain at least 50° to 70° of dorsiflexion.

(resection) arthroplasty."[15] However, each of these early studies suffers from a lack of outcomes measures. In a retrospective review of 58 patients, Hattrup and Johnson reported that 27.6% of patients were not satisfied with the outcome of a dorsal cheilectomy and noted that failure rates were higher with end-stage disease (37.5%) when compared to patients that displayed mild hallux rigidus (15%).[6]

The majority of failures following dorsal cheilectomy are likely due to poor patient selection and improper technique. Because cheilectomy only reduces the mechanical impingement at the first MTP joint, pain may persist or increase in patients selected with midrange pain or loss of greater than 50% of the articular cartilage of the first metatarsal head. It is these patients that would be better served with a first MTP arthrodesis. From a technical standpoint, as Shurnas and Coughlin have pointed out, many of the failures of cheilectomy in the literature have centered on "inadequate bony resection."[16] It has been their contention that a simple resection of the bony exostosis made flush with the dorsal cortex of the first metatarsal is inadequate. They have argued, therefore, that a proper resection should remove the dorsal 30% to 40% of the first metatarsal head.

Coughlin and Shurnas performed dorsal cheilectomies on 80 patients (93 feet) with hallux rigidus.[4] Their surgical technique involved resecting the dorsal, medial, and lateral osteophytes, along with resection of the dorsal 25% to 33% of the first metatarsal head. At a mean follow-up of 9.6 years, visual analog pain scores had significantly decreased from a mean score of 8 preoperatively to a mean score of 1.5

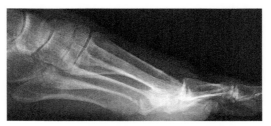

Fig. 8. Postoperative standing lateral radiograph demonstrating appropriate bony resection.

postoperatively, and patients were noted to have an increase in mean first MTP dorsiflexion from 14.5° preoperatively to 39° postoperatively. Mann and colleagues reported 85% pain relief, mean postoperative dorsiflexion of 30°, and minimal progression of arthrosis in a cohort of 20 patients undergoing dorsal cheilectomy.[2] In a retrospective review, Mann and Clanton reported a mean increase in postoperative range of motion of 19°, and 90% complete or significant pain relief. In this same study, 74% of patients demonstrated an improvement in total range of motion, whereas 16% demonstrated no improvement and 10% slightly less range of motion of the first MTP joint postoperatively.[1]

Successful results have been reported in both older patients and within the younger, more athletic population. In a study conducted by Feltham and colleagues, patients aged older than 60 years reported higher satisfaction rates postoperatively and demonstrated significantly higher American Orthopaedic Foot and Ankle Society (AOFAS) scores when compared to patients aged younger than 60 years.[17] Moreover, Mulier and colleagues examined the results of dorsal cheilectomy in high-level athletes with a mean age of 31 years and mean follow-up duration of 5.1 years.[7] In this study, they found that 75% of their patients were able to return to their prior level or high level of sports activity, with only 2 of the patients unable to return to their prior level attributing the dysfunction to the hallux. Functionally, 95% (21 out of 22) of the operative feet were rated as good or excellent in terms of first MTP motion, shoewear difficulties, and pain with activities.

Despite the universally positive results following dorsal cheilectomy, Rajan and colleagues demonstrated the inherent difficulty in predicting which patients would have a successful result. In this study, the authors noted statistically significant improvements between preoperative and postoperative Patient-reported Outcomes Measurement Information System (PROMIS) physical function, pain interference, and pain intensity scores. However, the preoperative PROMIS scores in patients undergoing a dorsal cheilectomy were not associated with preoperative to postoperative improvements in terms of the minimal clinically important difference.[18]

CLOSING

Dorsal cheilectomy remains a viable option for the patient with debilitating hallux rigidus, despite appropriate nonsurgical treatment modalities. It should be considered as a first-line surgical treatment option because it is relatively simple to perform, retains first MTP joint range of motion, is associated with a low rate of complications, and has been uniformly successful when an adequate bony resection is performed.

CLINICS CARE POINTS

- Capsular incision at least 5 mm medial to the EHL tendon to avoid violation of the tendon and to retain adequate capsular tissue for final closure at the end of the case.
- Resect dorsal osteophyte, along with 25% to 33% of the first metatarsal head. Avoid resecting more than this amount to decrease the chances of developing instability.
- Resect "kissing" osteophyte off of the dorsal base of the proximal phalanx.
- Strive to achieve at least 50° of passive dorsiflexion through the first MTP joint after cheilectomy. Consider addition of a Moberg osteotomy in cases where this level of dorsiflexion is not achieved.[10,11]
- Early patient-directed dorsiflexion and plantarflexion range of motion is essential to achieving a satisfactory result.

DISCLOSURE

I have no commercial or financial conflicts of interest to disclose about this article. In addition, no funding source to report (no funding provided).

REFERENCES

1. Mann RA, Clanton TO. Hallux rigidus: treatment by cheilectomy. J Bone Joint Surg Am 1988;70(3):400–6.
2. Mann RA, Coughlin MJ, DuVries HL. Hallux rigidus: a review of the literature and a method of treatment. Clin Orthop Relat Res 1979;142:57–63.
3. Nilsonne H. Hallux rigidus and its treatment. Acta Orthop Scand 1930;1:295–303.
4. Coughlin MJ, Shurnas PS. Hallux rigidus. Grading and long-term results of operative treatment. J Bone Joint Surg Am 2003;85(11):2072–88.
5. Harrison T, Fawzy E, Dinah F, et al. Prospective assessment of dorsal cheilectomy for hallux rigidus using a patient-reported outcome score. J Foot Ankle Surg 2010;49:232–7.
6. Hattrup SJ, Johnson KA. Subjective results of hallux rigidus following treatment with cheilectomy. Clin Orthop Relat Res 1988;226:182–91.
7. Mulier T, Steenwerckx A, Thienpont E, et al. Results after cheilectomy in athletes with hallux rigidus. Foot Ankle Int 1999;20(4):232–7.
8. Easley ME, Davis WH, Anderson RB. Intermediate to long-term follow-up of medial-approach dorsal cheilectomy for hallux rigidus. Foot Ankle Int 1999;20: 147–52.
9. Teoh KH, Tan WT, Atiyah Z, et al. Clinical outcomes following minimally invasive dorsal cheilectomy for hallux rigidus. Foot Ankle Int 2019;40(2):195–201.
10. Hamid KS, Parekh SG. Clinical presentation and management of hallux rigidus. Foot Ankle Clin 2015;20(3):391–9.
11. Thomas PJ, Smith RW. Proximal phalanx osteotomy for the surgical treatment of hallux rigidus. Foot Ankle Int 1999;20(1):3–12.
12. Razik A, Sott AH. Cheilectomy for hallux rigidus. Foot Ankle Clin 2016;21(3): 451–7.
13. Blair MP, Brown LA. Hallux limitus/rigidus deformity: a new great toe implant. J Foot Ankle Surg 1993;32(3):257–62.
14. Durrant MN, Siepert KK. Role of soft tissue structures as an etiology of hallux limitus. J Am Podiatr Med Assoc 1993;83(4):173–80.
15. Bonney G, Macnab I. Hallux valgus and hallux rigidus: a critical survey of operative results. J Bone Joint Surg Br 1952;34-B:366–85.
16. Shurnas PS, Coughlin MJ. Arthritic conditions of the foot. In: Coughlin MJ, Mann RA, Saltzman CL, editors. Surgery of the foot and ankle. 8th edition. Philadelphia: Mosby Elsevier; 2007. p. 805–921.
17. Feltham GT, Hanks SE, Marcus RE. Age-based outcomes of cheilectomy for the treatment of hallux rigidus. Foot Ankle Int 2001;22(3):192–7.
18. Rajan L, Conti MS, Cororaton A, et al. Relationship between preoperative PROMIS scores and postoperative outcomes in hallux rigidus patients undergoing cheilectomy. Foot Ankle Int 2022;43(8):1053–61.

Moberg and Moberg-Akin ('Mo-Akin') Osteotomies for Hallux Rigidus

Mohamad Issa, MD[a], Conor O'Neill, MD[a], Karl Schweitzer, MD[a,b,*]

KEYWORDS

- Hallux rigidus • Moberg osteotomy • Moberg-Akin osteotomy • Cheilectomy

KEY POINTS

- Hallux rigidus is a degenerative arthritis affecting the first metatarsophalangeal joint resulting in limited joint dorsiflexion during the early stages of the disease.
- Moberg osteotomy is a joint-sparing dorsal wedge osteotomy performed for early stages of hallux rigidus compensating the limited dorsiflexion with the preserved plantarflexion motion.
- Moberg osteotomy can be combined with Akin osteotomy creating a biplanar correction for hallux interphalangeus along with hallux rigidus.
- Moberg osteotomy results in overall high patient satisfaction with improvements in pain relief, function, and mobility in limited cohort and case series studies with absence of high-quality evidence studies.
- The reported complication rates of Moberg osteotomy are generally low and include nonunion, malunion, symptomatic hardware, soft tissue issues, and infection.

INTRODUCTION/BACKGROUND

Hallux rigidus represents a wide-spectrum of degenerative arthritis affecting the first metatarsophalangeal (MTP) joint. In the early disease stage, osteophytes and chondral wear are typically confined to the dorsal aspect of the joint, associated with limited dorsiflexion with preserved plantarflexion, and symptoms are limited to the late stance phase of the gait cycle, where first MTP joint dorsiflexion is necessary for the smooth transition to the pre-swing phase.[1] Historically, various treatment modalities have been proposed to limit disease progression and preserve joint range of motion. The most common joint-sparing procedure utilized has been the dorsal hallux cheilectomy.[2]

The desire to improve dorsiflexion motion (ie, beyond that of a cheilectomy) combined with early issues with joint-sacrificing procedures, such as the Keller resection

[a] Department of Orthopaedic Surgery, Duke University Medical Center, 311 Trent Drive, Durham, NC 27710, USA; [b] Foot and Ankle, 3480 Wake Forest Road, Suite 204, Raleigh, NC 27609, USA
* Corresponding author. 3480 Wake Forest Road, Suite 204, Raleigh, NC 27609.
E-mail address: karl.schweitzer@duke.edu

Foot Ankle Clin N Am 29 (2024) 425–442
https://doi.org/10.1016/j.fcl.2024.02.007
1083-7515/24/© 2024 Elsevier Inc. All rights reserved.

arthroplasty (eg, instability, cock-up toe deformity, transfer metatarsalgia) and hallux MTP joint arthrodesis (eg, malunion, nonunion), provided the impetus to develop a joint-sparing procedure with less potential for complications.[2] A uniplanar, proximal phalangeal, dorsiflexion-producing osteotomy for adolescents was first described in 1959 by Kessel and Bonney.[3] Moberg[4] later reported on his outcomes using this type of proximal phalangeal, dorsal closing wedge osteotomy in 8 adult patients and the procedure later became an eponymous term. Moberg proposed taking part of the preserved plantarflexion motion of the MTP joint to help accommodate the limited joint extension. This basic principle is a dorsal closing wedge osteotomy along the proximal phalanx base (**Fig. 1**). A biomechanical study by Kim and colleagues[5] demonstrated that Moberg osteotomy changes the center of pressure to a more plantar location of the proximal phalanx. This allows for load distribution to the healthier, plantar aspect of the joint, unloading the dorsal joint. This procedure was used with good success in combination with dorsal hallux cheilectomy for patients with varying degrees of hallux rigidus, lacking adequate dorsiflexion.[6,7]

A biplanar osteotomy method was later described and utilized for patients with hallux rigidus and mild hallux valgus or hallux interphalangeus, as a means of decompressing the dorsal and dorsolateral joint, improving relative dorsiflexion motion, and improving alignment to the hallux.[8,9] This type of biplanar proximal phalangeal osteotomy was performed in patients with moderate hallux rigidus and hallux valgus/interphalangeus and combined the dorsal closing wedge aspect of Moberg osteotomy with the medial closing wedge component of Akin osteotomy.[10] It was completed in conjunction with dorsal hallux cheilectomy, fixated with a cannulated compression screw, and performed through a dorsal or dorsomedial hallux MTP joint incision.[8,9] This procedure has become known as Moberg-Akin osteotomy or more concisely, a 'Mo-Akin.'

INDICATIONS

In general, surgery is indicated once the patient has undergone an adequate period of conservative treatment, generally greater than 6 months, including activity and

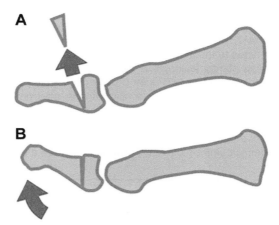

Fig. 1. (*A*) Diagram showing the dorsal wedge of Moberg osteotomy, with a dorsal base width usually around 2 to 4 mm (*B*) The osteotomy site reduced using a dorsiflexion force. (*From* Hazibullah Waizy, M. Abbara Czardybon, Stukenborg-Colsman C, et al. Mid- and long-term results of the joint preserving therapy of hallux rigidus. Archives of Orthopedic and Trauma Surgery. 2009;130(2):165-170. doi:https://doi.org/10.1007/s00402-009-0857-1)

shoewear modifications, orthotic use (eg, Morton's extension or turf toe plate), nonsteroidal anti-inflammatory drugs, and corticosteroid injection, without resolution of their symptoms.[5] More specifically, Moberg-Akin osteotomy combined with dorsal hallux cheilectomy is indicated for patients with symptomatic grade 2 or 3 hallux rigidus combined with hallux interphalangeus greater than 10°. It must be emphasized that Moberg osteotomy works best in patients with intact hallux MTP joint plantarflexion to compensate for deficient dorsiflexion. This relative shifting in the arc of hallux MTP joint motion with unloading of the arthritic dorsal joint and loading of the intact plantar joint can help limit the progression of the hallux rigidus disease.[11] The indications for Moberg osteotomy are the same as for Moberg-Akin osteotomy, except that the hallux should be normally aligned without significant hallux interphalangeus deformity (ie, <10°).

To better understand our specific indications for Moberg/Moberg-Akin osteotomy, it can be useful to know when we indicate patients for isolated dorsal hallux cheilectomy and arthrodesis procedures. We recommend dorsal hallux cheilectomy alone for symptomatic patients with (1) grades 1 through 3 hallux rigidus without significantly limited dorsiflexion (ie, Moberg/Moberg-Akin osteotomy not needed) and (2) grade 2 or 3 hallux rigidus with limited dorsiflexion and plantarflexion (ie, not adequate plantarflexion for patient to benefit from osteotomy). A hallux MTP joint arthrodesis is recommended for symptomatic patients with (1) severe grade 4 hallux rigidus changes and (2) grade 3 or 4 hallux rigidus with moderate to severe hallux valgus deformity.

CONTRAINDICATIONS

The specific contraindications for this procedure are primarily related to the biomechanics of this osteotomy, as highlighted in the prior section. A requirement for the osteotomy to be effective is limited joint dorsiflexion with preserved plantarflexion. In a patient with hallux rigidus with preserved dorsiflexion and plantarflexion, Moberg-Akin osteotomy has limited ability to effect a change to the biomechanics of the joint. Conversely, in a patient with hallux rigidus with limited dorsiflexion and plantarflexion, the mechanics of the osteotomy are not favorable. Thus, the contraindications for Moberg-Akin osteotomy include (1) intact hallux MTP dorsiflexion, (2) impaired hallux MTP plantarflexion, (3) grade 4 hallux rigidus, (4) normal hallux MTP joint alignment, (5) active infection or open wound at intended surgical site, and (6) comorbidities that would otherwise contraindicate the patient for a forefoot reconstructive surgery.

Moberg/Moberg-AKIN ('Mo-AKIN) SURGICAL TECHNIQUE
Preoperative Planning

- A through physical examination is required to appreciate the MTP joint range of motion. The extent of both dorsiflexion and plantarflexion needs to be determined (**Fig. 2**).
  - It is important that the patient be aware that the benefit of additional dorsiflexion will be from the relative loss of some plantarflexion of the hallux MTP joint.
- Four-view weight-bearing foot radiographs (including sesamoid view) (**Fig. 3**)
  - Lateral foot radiograph allows for visualization of dorsal hallux MTP joint osteophytes and joint space narrowing.
  - Anteroposterior foot radiograph to evaluate the extent of hallux MTP joint arthritis and hallux alignment, specifically for the latter, to evaluate for hallux valgus (or varus) and hallux interphalangeal deformity. Keep in mind that

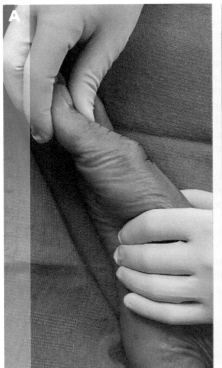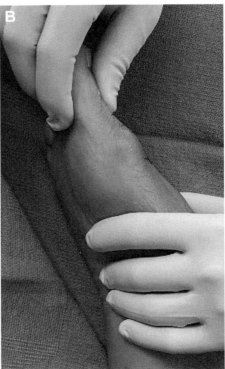

Fig. 2. Intraoperative photograph demonstrating preoperative range of motion (*A*: plantar-flexion, *B*:dorsiflexion) of the hallux metatarsophalangeal (MTP) joint. In this patient with hallux rigidus, there is preserved plantarflexion and limited dorsiflexion, which serves as a good indication for performing Moberg/Moberg-Akin osteotomy as an addition to dorsal hallux cheilectomy.

extensive dorsal osteophytosis can impair overall hallux MTP joint visualization and overestimate the extent of joint-space narrowing.
○ Sesamoid view can allow for the detection of any sesamoid-first metatarsal arthritis and evaluate the extent of first metatarsal rotation, particularly in relationship to any existing hallux valgus deformity.

Operating Room Preparation

- Regional (ie, ultrasound-guided popliteal-saphenous nerve block) and monitored anesthesia care are typically utilized.
- The patient is positioned supine with a rolled blanket 'bump' under the hip to allow for neutral foot positioning during the case.
- A well-padded thigh tourniquet is applied. In our experience, an ankle esmarch tourniquet can preferentially impact the foot and ankle flexor tendons, which can prevent accurate intraoperative range of motion assessments.
- Preoperative intravenous antibiotic, typically 2g Ancef (cefazolin), and a single dose of tranexamic acid are given prior to the incision to limit bleeding and optimize postoperative wound healing.
- Intraoperative mini-C arm fluoroscopy is required during the procedure.

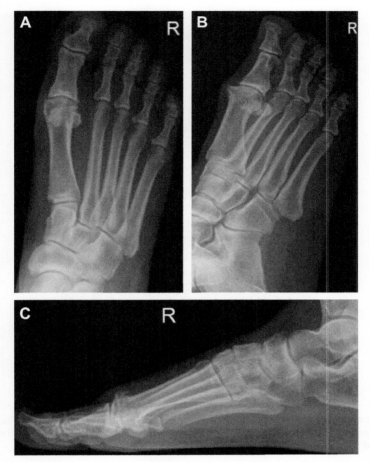

Fig. 3. Preoperative weight-bearing radiographs views of the foot (*A*: anteroposterior, *B*: oblique, *C*: lateral) of patient shown in **Fig. 2**, demonstrating moderate hallux rigidus changes and hallux valgus/interphalangeus deformity.

Approach

- A short, dorsal incision is marked out, centered over the hallux MTP joint and made slightly medial to the medial border of the extensor hallucis longus (EHL) tendon (**Fig. 4**).
- The choice of a dorsal incision is utilitarian, particularly in the case of an eventual need for conversion to a hallux MTP joint arthrodesis if symptomatic, more global joint arthritis develops.
- Moberg originally described an S-shaped dorsal incision, which is less commonly performed today. The procedure can also be performed through a dorsomedial or medial approach, depending on the associated procedures or surgeon preference.
- A dorsal incision is made, followed by a longitudinal hallux MTP arthrotomy, which is made medial to the EHL tendon. The EHL tendon is mobilized and retracted laterally. It is critical to protect the EHL tendon throughout the case.

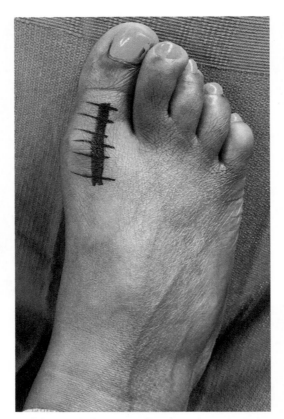

Fig. 4. Intraoperative photograph showing a dorsal incision centered over the hallux meta-tarsophalangeal (MTP) joint. Hallux valgus/interphalangeus is appreciated with the hallux positioned slightly under the second toe.

Medial and lateral arthrotomy flaps are carefully raised proximally around the metatarsal head and distally at the proximal phalanx, to expose the joint, along with impinging dorsal osteophytes on both sides of the joint.

- The dorsomedial nerve of the hallux, while not routinely visualized during the case, is protected throughout the procedure, particularly while elevating the medial arthrotomy.
- Two Senn retractors or a self-retaining retractor is used to maintain the needed exposure (**Fig. 5**).
- Hyperflexion of the hallux MTP joint allows for complete visualization of the articular cartilage on both sides of the joint. Intact plantar joint cartilage is critical for the success of Moberg-Akin osteotomy.
- Thorough joint inspection allows for intraoperative decision-making on the most optimal procedure. This includes assessment of viability of performing Moberg/Moberg-Akin osteotomy in addition to dorsal hallux cheilectomy, but also on potential conversion to an arthrodesis, should more global arthritis be present. Thus, appropriate preoperative counseling and discussion should be held with the patient in borderline cases, to allow for intraoperative decision-making on the most optimal procedure to be performed.

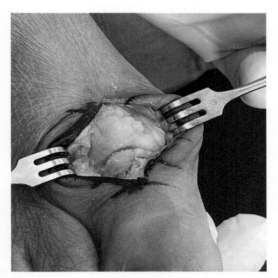

Fig. 5. Intraoperative photograph showing the exposed hallux metatarsophalangeal (MTP) joint using 2 Senn retractors. The extensor hallucis longus (EHL) tendon and lateral capsule are retracted; lateral and medial capsule and dorsomedial nerve of hallux retracted medially.

Dorsal Hallux Cheilectomy

- A microsagittal saw blade (size: 9 mm wide x 25 mm long) is utilized for osteophyte resection on both the metatarsal and phalangeal sides of the joint. Appropriate retraction of the soft tissues is critical, along with the use of saline irrigation to prevent thermal necrosis. We typically use a 2-cut technique on the dorsal hallux metatarsal head side, starting with a flat cut, followed by a dorsally angulated cut.
- Following cheilectomy, the joint is manually manipulated into dorsiflexion and plantarflexion to help break up any residual scarring and improve motion. In addition, a Freer elevator can be used to carefully free up any adhesions between the plantar metatarsal head and sesamoid complex.
- The medial and lateral edges are beveled smooth using a small rongeur and/or microsagittal saw (**Fig. 6**).
- Around 20% to 30% of the metatarsal head can be removed without the risk of destabilizing the joint.[12]
- If dorsal hallux cheilectomy fails to produce dorsiflexion beyond 70°, it is recommended to perform Moberg/Moberg-Akin osteotomy.[13] In the case of a patient having dorsiflexion beyond 70° following cheilectomy, there is less opportunity for Moberg/Moberg-Akin osteotomy to provide additional benefit to the patient, unless specific patient factors necessitate it (eg, a dancer/ballerina) (**Fig. 7**).
- A minimally invasive approach using a Shannon burr and standard technique can be utilized to potentially reduce stiffness and healing time.

Moberg Osteotomy

- Additional exposure is made to the dorsal aspect of the proximal phalangeal base for site of intended osteotomy completion.

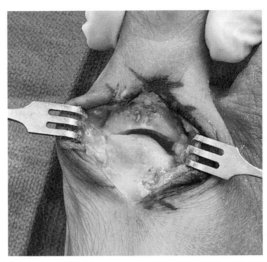

Fig. 6. Intraoperative photograph showing the decompressed metatarsophalangeal (MTP) joint after dorsal hallux cheilectomy.

- For either osteotomy choice, a 0.045 Kirschner wire is placed dorsally at the center of the intended osteotomy and fluoroscopy is used to confirm appropriate wire location. It is critical to ensure that there is adequate space to perform and fixate the planned osteotomy, to avoid being intraarticular and to avoid hardware prominence.

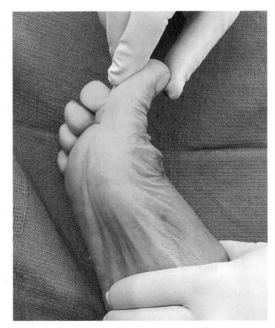

Fig. 7. Intraoperative photograph demonstrating around 60° of maximal dorsiflexion of the hallux metatarsophalangeal (MTP) joint following cheilectomy, which represents a good indication for performing Moberg/Moberg-Akin osteotomy.

- To achieve maximal dorsiflexion effect, the osteotomy should be as proximal as possible.[14] As noted earlier, adequate proximal bone is required for the fixation method and to prevent fracture of the proximal fragment.
- Using a microsagittal saw blade (size: 7 mm wide x 18.5 mm long), the first osteotomy cut is made along the dorsal wire, which serves as a guide. Care is taken to not violate the plantar cortex of the proximal phalanx. Once the osteotomy direction has been determined the wire can be removed. We prefer to make the initial cut essentially parallel to the MTP joint axis.
- The second cut is completed around 2 to 4 mm distal to the first cut, depending on the extent of correction needed. While the cut is directed proximally to create the dorsal wedge, it remains parallel otherwise to the first cut. We generally recommend starting with less wedge osteotomy thickness than is considered necessary and then fine tuning the correction gradually. To do this, we manually close the osteotomy while running the microsagittal saw blade within the osteotomy site. This can avoid taking a larger resection than desired and help 'dial in' the exact correction needed.
  - In a neutrally aligned hallux, it is critical that the 2 cuts be parallel in the anteroposterior plane (ie, only angulated in the lateral plane) to avoid introducing any valgus or varus deformity to the toe (**Fig. 8**).
- The proximal phalanx can now be gently dorsiflexed to close the dorsal wedge and reduce the osteotomy. If the osteotomy is not closing as desired, we carefully run the microsagittal saw within the osteotomy to remove any osseous irregularities that may be blocking the reduction. These 'high points' generally occur at the medial and lateral cortices. If the osteotomy was not carried plantar enough, this can also prevent appropriate reduction, in which case, the saw blade is used to complete a bit more of the osteotomy plantarly.

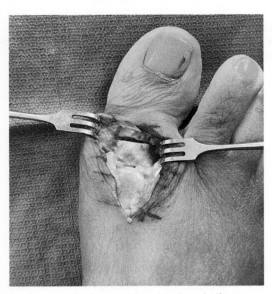

Fig. 8. Intraoperative photograph showing dorsal hallux cheilectomy and Moberg osteotomy prior to reduction and fixation. Note the parallel osteotomy cuts in the anteroposterior plane.

'Mo-Akin' (Moberg-Akin Osteotomy)

- The 'Mo-Akin' osteotomy is commonly performed for hallux rigidus in the setting of hallux interphalangeus in which a biplanar correction is needed.
- The same surgical approach is made as for Moberg osteotomy.
- The initial cut over a guide wire is performed as per the Moberg osteotomy technique.
- The second cut is be performed 2 to 4 mm distal and angulated both proximally and laterally creating a dorsomedial, biplanar wedge.
- The dorsomedial wedge can be removed and osteotomy reduced, creating the necessary correction in 2 planes.
- For the reduction, the toe should be dorsiflexed along with application of a varus force to close down the biplanar osteotomy.
- A minimally invasive approach can also be utilized for either Moberg or Moberg-Akin osteotomy and fixated with a headless screw placed over a guidewire. This may have the potential benefit of reduced postoperative swelling and healing times.

Osteotomy Fixation

- Multiple fixation methods have been proposed to stabilize and compress the osteotomy site, including cerclage wire, screw, Kirschner wires, compression staple, mini-plate with screws, and other options, such as a plate-staple combination (eg, Plaple, Arthrex, Inc).
- The fixation method used initially by Moberg included a stainless steel wire run between 2 drill holes along both sides of the dorsal osteotomy. The wire limbs are twisted for osteotomy compression and the cut wire ends are buried in 1 of the burr holes[4] (**Fig. 9**).
  - This is a cost-effective method; however, there can be concerns with wire cutout, adequate osteotomy compression for healing, and prominent hardware.
- Fixation with a Kirschner wire is cost-effective as well.
  - This technique can be associated with possible loss of reduction, lack of active compression across the osteotomy, and infection.

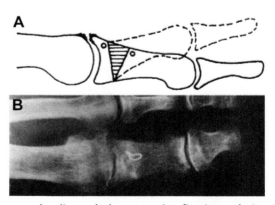

Fig. 9. (*A, B*) Diagram and radiograph demonstrating fixation technique described by Moberg using a wire through 2 dorsal drill holes. (*From* MOBERG E. A Simple Operation for Hallux Rigidus. Clinical Orthopedics and Related Research. 1979;(142):55-56. doi:https://doi.org/10.1097/00003086-197907000-00009)

- The Plaple (Arthrex, Inc, plate with a staple component) is another option that provides good stability and fixation (**Fig. 10**). It is associated with higher costs than earlier fixation methods highlighted earlier.
- The preferred fixation method by the author is a single dorsal nitinol staple (Arthrex DynaNite nitinol staple, size 11W x 10L)
  - This method is both reliable and fast, but also has associated higher costs.
  - The staple is composed of nitinol and provides the benefit of continuous compression for osteotomy healing.
  - It is vital to position the compression staple perpendicular to the osteotomy to maximize compression and stability, along with centering the staple over the reduced osteotomy to avoid implant leg cutout.
  - It is placed using the standard technique (**Fig. 11**).

Final Technique Points and Postoperative Recovery

- The hallux proximal phalanx is tested along the MTP range of motion arc (**Fig. 12**). Hunt and Anderson[9] also recommended in their retrospective series of Moberg-Akin osteotomies as a guide, that the plantar aspect of the hallux should sit about 3 to 5 mm off of a flat plate used during surgery to gauge the degree of dorsiflexion.
- Final fluoroscopic views are taken to assure the appropriate correction is obtained with Moberg/Moberg-Akin osteotomy and to confirm osteotomy reduction and hardware placement (**Figs. 13** and **14**).
- The tourniquet is released, and hemostasis is achieved using Bovie electrocautery.
- The surgical wound and hallux MTP joint are thoroughly irrigated out.
- The hallux MTP joint capsule is closed using interrupted 2-0 Vicryl suture.
- The dermal layer is closed using 3-0 Vicryl suture.
- The skin is approximated using 3-0 Monocryl and skin glue (**Fig. 15**).
- Once the glue is dry, the incision is covered using Xeroform, followed by 4 × 4 gauze, soft padding, and elastic bandage wrap.
- The patient is placed in a hard sole postoperative shoe, allowed to be weight-bearing as tolerated, and encouraged to perform early hallux MTP joint range of motion once the surgical dressings are removed around 7 to 10 days postoperatively. Goal is for the patient to wear a supportive tennis shoe by 4 to 6 weeks with unrestricted, full activity by 3 months postoperatively.

COMPLICATIONS

Moberg/Moberg-Akin osteotomies are variations of proximal phalangeal osteotomy that are often performed in conjunction with other procedures, such as dorsal hallux

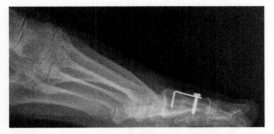

Fig. 10. Postoperative radiograph showing a cheilectomy and healed Moberg osteotomy using the Plaple implant. (*From* Warganich T, Harris T. Moberg Osteotomy for Hallux Rigidus. Foot and Ankle Clinics. 2015;20(3):433-450. doi:https://doi.org/10.1016/j.fcl.2015.04.006)

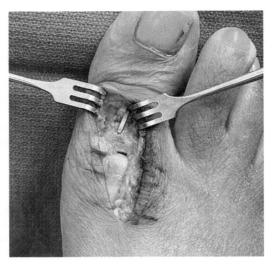

Fig. 11. Intraoperative photograph demonstrating dorsal Moberg-Akin osteotomy fixation using a nitinol staple.

cheilectomy. This osteotomy is rarely done in isolation, thus there is little literature on the specific rates of complications associated with it done in isolation. As for all periarticular osteotomies done throughout the body, standard complications include nonunion, malunion, hardware pain, wound issues, and infections. That being said, the relative complication rates with this procedure are generally very low.

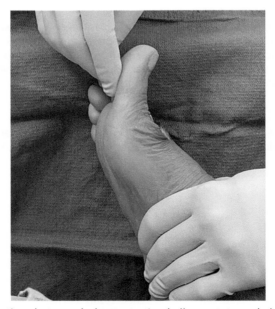

Fig. 12. Intraoperative photograph demonstrating hallux metatarsophalangeal joint dorsiflexion after Moberg osteotomy, which is around 85°.

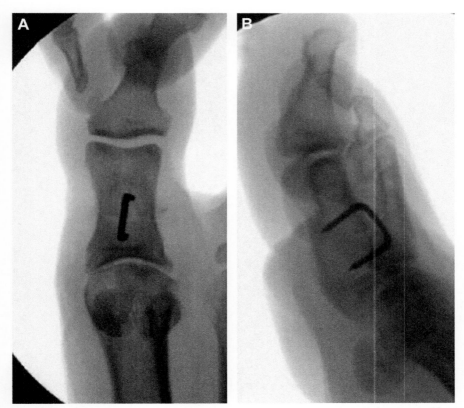

Fig. 13. Intraoperative (*A*: anteroposterior and *B*: lateral) fluoroscopic images showing a Moberg-Akin osteotomy fixated with a nitinol compression staple.

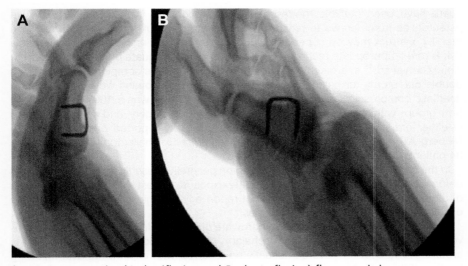

Fig. 14. Intraoperative (*A*: dorsiflexion and *B*: plantarflexion) fluoroscopic images.

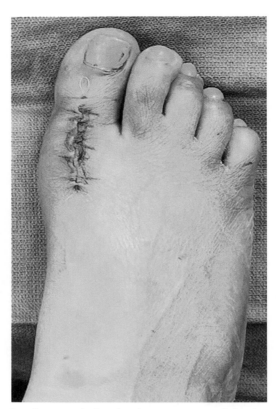

Fig. 15. Intraoperative photograph showing foot appearance following a Moberg-Akin osteotomy and dorsal hallux cheilectomy.

Nonunion, Malunion, and Symptomatic Hardware

There have been multiple modes of fixation suggested for Moberg/Moberg-Akin osteotomies from screws to tensioned wire to staples, but no convincing evidence that 1 construct may be superior in preventing nonunion or malunion. Overall, this risk is rare if appropriate technique is carried out and adequate osteotomy compression is achieved.[15] In a recent study of 74 Akin osteotomies completed as a part of a double osteotomy for hallux valgus correction, 39 osteotomies were fixated with a headless compression screw and 35 with a staple. There was a 100% union rate in both groups with no cases of fixation failure, no revision surgery, and no delayed union in either group.[16] Hunt and Anderson[9] retrospectively reported on a series of 35 Moberg-Akin osteotomies combined with dorsal hallux cheilectomies performed in 34 patients. All biplanar osteotomies healed.

In the case of Moberg osteotomy, malunion generally presents as a varus or valgus deformity and has been linked to inadequate exposure to best visualize the parallelism of the cuts.[6] Hunt and Anderson[9] did not report any malunions in their retrospective case series on Moberg-Akin osteotomies.

There is also a risk of symptomatic hardware given the relatively thin, soft tissue envelope that surrounds the proximal phalanx. Symptomatic hardware prevalence is around 3% to 8%.[17,18] This can usually be resolved with implant removal following healing of the osteotomy.[17]

Soft Tissues

It is also important to recognize the deeper soft tissue structures that are at risk with osteotomy. Deliberate care must be taken to protect the EHL, flexor hallucis longus, and dorsomedial cutaneous nerve, which are all nearby structures at risk.[7]

Infection

Infection rates are reported as very low with either Moberg or Moberg-Akin osteotomy. Kilmartin and colleagues[18] reported no infections in his series of 49 Moberg osteotomies. O'Malley and colleagues[17] reported an infection rate of 1% with 81 Moberg osteotomies. Hunt and Anderson[9] had 1 patient with a mild wound dehiscence that required some local wound care to heal completely.

Secondary Metatarsalgia and Interphalangeal Arthritis

Due to changes in the natural biomechanics and offloading of the distal aspect of the first ray, patients undergoing Moberg/Moberg-Akin osteotomy can develop a secondary metatarsalgia, which generally presents at the plantar first or second metatarsal head. O'Malley and colleagues[17] reported a 1% incidence of this secondary metatarsalgia. Eight percent (4/49) of patients in a prospective study by Kilmartin and colleagues[18] presented in the postoperative period with secondary metatarsalgia.

The biomechanical effect of Moberg/Moberg-Akin osteotomy shifts the location of the contact pressure seen at the MTP joint plantarly, but other secondary effects can be seen with overload of the interphalangeal joint and resulting adjacent joint arthritis.[5] In a study by Chrea and colleagues,[19] 1.4% of Moberg osteotomy patients (1/73) developed symptomatic arthritis at the hallux interphalangeal joint. Kilmartin and colleagues[18] demonstrated a 6% (3/49) incidence of hallux interphalangeal arthritis.

Persistent/Recurrent Pain and Revision Surgery

Chrea and colleagues[19] discussed an 11% incidence (8/73) of persistent pain and symptoms at the hallux MTP joint following Moberg osteotomy and dorsal hallux cheilectomy. Kilmartin and colleagues[18] similarly reported a 10% incidence (3/49) of patients with persistent pain in the MTP joint. Revisions of Moberg/Moberg-Akin osteotomies, while not common, mostly include conversion to hallux MTP joint arthrodesis for continued pain.[17] Converting Moberg/Moberg-Akin osteotomy and dorsal hallux cheilectomy to arthrodesis can be difficult due to the increased relative extension of the proximal phalanx, which can make the use of a precontoured MTP arthrodesis plate difficult, and may lead to excessive dorsiflexion positioning of the hallux MTP joint arthrodesis.[20]

CLINICAL OUTCOMES

Most of the literature on outcomes of Moberg/Moberg-Akin osteotomies is from smaller case series and cohorts with favorable results, without substantial high-level data to support it. While a broad look at the literature suggests that Moberg/Moberg-Akin osteotomy and dorsal hallux cheilectomy can work well together for select patients with painful hallux rigidus who have failed conservative treatment, there is little high-quality evidence available.[13]

Blyth and colleagues[7] reported on their results of Moberg osteotomies at a mean of 4 years follow-up, and patients showed an 83% (15/18) improvement, with good to excellent results in 77% (14/18). One patient in this series had persisting pain and required a subsequent arthrodesis. Thomas and colleagues[6] found an overall satisfaction rate of 96% without complication or revision in their retrospective review of 17 patients treated with Moberg osteotomy at a mean 2.5-year follow-up. O'Malley and colleagues[17] performed a similar retrospective analysis of 81 patients with hallux rigidus, reporting an 85% satisfaction rate after Moberg osteotomy and dorsal hallux cheilectomy. Around 5% of patients (4/81) in their study did go on to require secondary conversion to hallux MTP joint arthrodesis due to persisting pain. In a prospective study by Kilmartin and colleagues,[18] 89% of patients were overall satisfied with the Moberg osteotomy procedure, with 65% of patients completely satisfied, 24% satisfied with reservation, and 11% dissatisfied.

In an isolated report of Moberg osteotomies performed without cheilectomy, Citron and colleagues[15] reported on 10 cases in 8 patients at a mean follow-up of 22 years with lasting results. Initially all patients had relief of symptoms, with 50% (5/10) remaining symptom free at final follow-up. Four patients had pain with the ambulation and 1 patient required conversion to arthrodesis.[15]

Waizy and colleagues[21] published a prospective study of 60 patients in which 33 patients underwent Moberg osteotomy, performed specifically in cases where dorsiflexion was 70° or less after dorsal hallux cheilectomy. They found at a mean of 8 years follow-up, the majority of patients had continued pain relief and overall satisfaction, without the need for revision surgery. The results of a recent meta-analysis of 11 studies investigating 374 cases of Moberg osteotomy with cheilectomy showed revision rates were low at 4.8%, and overall patient satisfaction is high at 77% (288/374 cases).[13]

Hunt and Anderson,[9] in their retrospective case series of 35 Moberg-Akin osteotomies performed in combination with dorsal hallux cheilectomies in 34 patients at a mean follow-up of 22.5 months, found 90% of patients reported good to excellent results, with good pain relief, improved function, and less shoewear limitations. It should be noted that the majority of patients in this study had more advanced hallux rigidus, with 62% being grade 3 (19/34) or 4 (2/34) preoperatively.

Maes and colleagues,[22] in their prospective study of 105 feet undergoing dorsal hallux cheilectomy with Moberg-Akin osteotomy for grades 0 to 4 hallux rigidus (88% were either grade 2 or 3), found significant improvements in pain, function, quality of life, and hallux MTP joint mobility at the 12-month follow-up.[22–24] The reoperation rate reported at 14.3% at 12 months, was slightly higher than for other studies, and was mostly due to hardware pain and need for removal of staple used for osteotomy fixation.

CLINICS CARE POINTS

- Moberg and Moberg-Akin osteotomies are vital joint-sacrificing procedures for the treatment of early stages of hallux rigidus and hallux interphalangeus.
- Inspection of articular cartilage on both sides of the joint is paramount as an intact plantar joint cartilage is critical for the success of Moberg/Moberg-Akin osteotomy.
- Surgeon should always be prepared to adjust the procedure required depending on the intraoperative findings which require appropriate preoperative counseling and discussion regarding possible joint arthrodesis.
- If the osteotomy is not closing as desired, carefully run the microsagittal saw within the osteotomy to remove any osseous irregularities that may be blocking the reduction which generally occur at the medial and lateral cortices.
- Moberg osteotomy can be combined with Akin osteotomy for hallux rigidus in the setting of hallux interphalangeus where a biplanar correction is needed.

- Single dorsal nitinol staple provides reliable and quick fixation to the osteotomy with the benefit of continuous compression for optimal healing.
- It is vital to position the compression staple perpendicular to the osteotomy to maximize compression and stability, along with centering the staple over the reduced osteotomy to avoid implant leg cutout.
- The osteotomy has rare complications including nonunion, malunion, wound issues, infection, and symptomatic hardware.
- The procedure has favorable outcomes and high patient satisfaction rates in small case series in the absence of high-quality evidence-based studies.

DISCLOSURE

The authors declare that they have no conflicts of interest or financial relationships that could influence the objectivity, integrity, or impartiality of the content presented.

REFERENCES

1. Allan JJ, McClelland JA, Munteanu SE, et al. First metatarsophalangeal joint range of motion is associated with lower limb kinematics in individuals with first metatarsophalangeal joint osteoarthritis. J Foot Ankle Res 2020;13(1):1–8.
2. Galois L, Hemmer J, Ray V, et al. Surgical options for hallux rigidus: state of the art and review of the literature. Eur J Orthop Surg Traumatol 2020;30:57–65.
3. Kessel L, Bonney G. Hallux rigidus in the adolescent. Journal of Bone and Joint Surgery British 1958;40(4):668–73.
4. MOBERG E. A simple operation for hallux rigidus. Clin Orthop Relat Res 1979; 142:55–6 (1976-2007).
5. Kim PH-U, Chen X, Hillstrom H, et al. Moberg osteotomy shifts contact pressure plantarly in the first metatarsophalangeal joint in a biomechanical model. Foot Ankle Int 2016;37(1):96–101.
6. Thomas PJ, Smith RW. Proximal phalanx osteotomy for the surgical treatment of hallux rigidus. Foot Ankle Int 1999;20(1):3–12.
7. Blyth M, Mackay D, Kinninmonth A. Dorsal wedge osteotomy in the treatment of hallux rigidus. J Foot Ankle Surg 1998;37(1):8–10.
8. Hunt KJ, Anderson RB. Biplanar oblique closing wedge osteotomy of the hallux proximal phalanx with screw fixation. Tech Foot Ankle Surg 2009;8(3):155–8.
9. Hunt KJ, Anderson RB. Biplanar proximal phalanx closing wedge osteotomy for hallux rigidus. Foot Ankle Int 2012;33(12):1043–50.
10. Akin O. The treatment of hallux valgus: a new operative procedure and its results. Med sentinel 1925;33:678–9.
11. Coughlin MJ, Shurnas PS. Hallux rigidus: grading and long-term results of operative treatment. JBJS 2003;85(11):2072–88.
12. Lau JT, Daniels TR. Outcomes following cheilectomy and interpositional arthroplasty in hallux rigidus. Foot Ankle Int 2001;22(6):462–70.
13. Roukis TS. Outcomes after cheilectomy with phalangeal dorsiflexory osteotomy for hallux rigidus: a systematic review. J Foot Ankle Surg 2010;49(5):479–87.
14. Seibert NR, Kadakia AR. Surgical management of hallux rigidus: cheilectomy and osteotomy (phalanx and metatarsal). Foot Ankle Clin 2009;14(1):9–22.
15. Citron N, Neil M. Dorsal wedge osteotomy of the proximal phalanx for hallux rigidus. Long-term results. Journal of Bone & Joint Surgery British 1987;69(5):835–7.

16. Fazal M, Simon H, Bacarese-Hamilton J, et al. Screw versus staple fixation for Akin osteotomy. Ann R Coll Surg Engl 2022;104(1):53–6.
17. O'Malley MJ, Basran HS, Gu Y, et al. Treatment of advanced stages of hallux rigidus with cheilectomy and phalangeal osteotomy. JBJS 2013;95(7):606–10.
18. Kilmartin TE. Phalangeal osteotomy versus first metatarsal decompression osteotomy for the surgical treatment of hallux rigidus: a prospective study of age-matched and condition-matched patients. J Foot Ankle Surg 2005;44(1):2–12.
19. Chrea B, Eble SK, Day J, et al. Comparison between polyvinyl alcohol implant and cheilectomy with Moberg osteotomy for hallux rigidus. Foot Ankle Int 2020;41(9):1031–40.
20. Ho B, Baumhauer J. Hallux rigidus. EFORT Open Reviews 2017;2(1):13–20.
21. Waizy H, Abbara Czardybon M, Stukenborg-Colsman C, et al. Mid-and long-term results of the joint preserving therapy of hallux rigidus. Arch Orthop Trauma Surg 2010;130:165–70.
22. Maes DJ, De Vil J, Kalmar AF, et al. Clinical and radiological outcomes of hallux rigidus treated with cheilectomy and a Moberg-Akin osteotomy. Foot Ankle Int 2020;41(3):294–302.
23. Waizy Hazibullah, Czardybon M Abbara, Stukenborg-Colsman C, et al. Mid- and long-term results of the joint preserving therapy of hallux rigidus. Arch Orthop Trauma Surg 2009;130(2):165–70.
24. Warganich T, Harris T. Moberg Osteotomy for Hallux Rigidus. Foot Ankle Clin 2015;20(3):433–50.

Interpositional Arthroplasty for Hallux Rigidus
Surgical Technique and Outcomes Discussion

Albert T. Anastasio, MD, Colleen Wixted, MD*,
James A. Nunley II, MD

KEYWORDS

- Hallux rigidus, • Interpositional arthroplasty, • Capsular interpositional arthroplasty,
- Cheilectomy, • Tendon interpositional arthroplasty,
- Modified oblique Keller capsular interpositional arthroplasty

KEY POINTS

- Interpositional arthroplasty options for hallux rigidus (HR) allow for maintenance of range of motion (ROM) at the metatarsophalangeal joint with the goal of improved pain and ROM through resection of the diseased articular surface.
- Capsular interpositional arthroplasty involves resection of metatarsophalangeal joint (MTPJ) capsular tissues, removal of dorsal osteophytosis, resection of diseased joint space, and suturing of the raised capsular flap to the plantar plate.
- Regardless of specific subtype, interpositional arthroplasty has demonstrated good clinical and functional outcomes. However, there is substantial heterogeneity about outcome reporting and surgical techniques for interpositional arthroplasty within the literature.

 Video content accompanies this article at http://www.foot.theclinics.com.

INTRODUCTION

Hallux rigidus (HR) is one of the most common pathologic conditions encountered by foot and ankle surgeons. Other articles in this unique series on HR have discussed pathophysiology, classification, presentation, diagnostic considerations, and treatment protocols for this condition. Surgical treatment options are broad, ranging from isolated cheilectomy in mild cases with primarily dorsal involvement to arthrodesis for end-stage HR, with complete joint involvement and angular or rotational deformity. Interpositional arthroplasty procedures for HR have demonstrated success in reducing pain while maintaining range of motion (ROM) at the metatarsophalangeal

Division of Foot and Ankle Surgery, Department of Orthopaedic Surgery, Duke University, 200 Trent Drive, Durham, NC 27710, USA
* Corresponding author.
E-mail address: Colleen.wixted@gmail.com

Foot Ankle Clin N Am 29 (2024) 443–454
https://doi.org/10.1016/j.fcl.2023.10.004
1083-7515/24/© 2023 Elsevier Inc. All rights reserved.

foot.theclinics.com

joint (MTPJ). However, these procedures are subject to failures including continued pain and MTPJ subluxation.

The purpose of this review is to focus specifically on interpositional arthroplasty options for HR. We will discuss technique considerations for interpositional arthroplasty and provide a literature review on the relative success of various interpositional arthroplasty subtypes.

Surgical Technique

We present here our technique for capsular interposition arthroplasty (Video 1). Although numerous techniques have been described for various forms of interpositional arthroplasty for HR, most approaches use a dorsal or a medial approach. We favor a dorsal approach, allowing for ease of access to the lateral osteophyte and capsular tissues.

Standard anteroposterior (AP) and lateral radiographs are obtained preoperatively (**Fig. 1**A and B). The patient is positioned supine with a bump under the contralateral hip to neutralize foot positioning. Prepping and draping is carried out following standard technique, and a miniature C-arm is used for the procedure. An Esmarch tourniquet at the ankle may be used to exsanguinate the foot. A longitudinal dorsal incision is carried out, approximately from the level of the interphalangeal joint to roughly 2 cm proximal to the MTPJ overlying the extensor hallucis longus (EHL) tendon (**Fig. 2**A). The dorsomedial sensory cutaneous branch of the superficial peroneal nerve is identified and is protected carefully throughout the procedure. The EHL tendon is identified and is carefully separated from the underlying extensor hallucis brevis (EHB) tendon. The EHL tendon is then mobilized and retracted laterally, and a capsular flap is raised from the proximal phalanx, taking care to ensure that as much capsular tissue as possible is lifted directly from the bone (see **Fig. 2**B). This tissue is reflected to the level of the MTPJ, and the joint is then carefully inspected.

On inspection of the joint, if greater than 50% of the articular surface seems nonarthritic, the surgeon may consider a native-joint salvage procedure such as isolated cheilectomy. If less than 50% of the articular surface remains, the patient is likely to

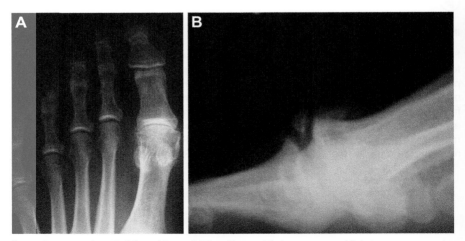

Fig. 1. Preoperative AP (*A*) and lateral (*B*) radiographic images reveal joint space narrowing and dorsal osteophytosis at the MTPJ. Of note, only very mild hallux valgus is appreciated and sesamoidal evaluation reveals absence of a significant pronation deformity.

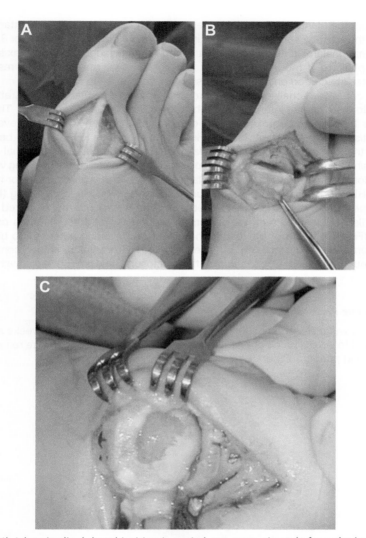

Fig. 2. (*A*) A longitudinal dorsal incision is carried out, approximately from the level of the interphalangeal joint to roughly 2 cm proximal to the MTPJ overlying the EHL tendon. (*B*) A capsular flap is raised from the proximal phalanx, taking care to ensure that as much capsular tissue as possible is lifted directly from the bone. This tissue is reflected to the level of the MTPJ, and the joint is then carefully inspected. (*C*) If less than 50% of the joint space remains (as in this case), the decision is made to proceed with cheilectomy and capsular interpositional arthroplasty in lieu of isolated dorsal cheilectomy.

remain symptomatic after isolated cheilectomy (see **Fig. 2**C). Thus, we favor proceeding with cheilectomy with interpositional arthroplasty. To expose the dorsal aspect of the distal metatarsal for cheilectomy, the capsular flap is carefully elevated proximately over the dorsal osteophytosis in a subperiosteal fashion. The dorsal osteophytes are carefully removed using either a sagittal saw or a rongeur. A McGlamry elevator can then be applied to release the plantar plate and flexor hallucis brevis tendon from the plantar aspect of the metatarsal. The great toe is then plantarflexed, revealing the articular surface at the proximal phalanx. Roughly one-fourth or 8 mm of the proximal phalanx is resected using a sagittal saw, orthogonally to the axis of the proximal phalanx. If more than roughly 25% of the proximal phalanx is resected, MTPJ instability can be encountered postoperatively.

Having completed cheilectomy and proximal phalanx articular resection, attention is turned to the capsular interposition arthroplasty portion of the procedure. The EHB tendon is transected approximately 3 cm proximal to the MTPJ to prevent the capsular tissue from being retracted during ambulation. The EHB can also be mobilized into the joint space with the capsular tissues to augment interpositional arthroplasty. Using nonabsorbable suture, the previously raised capsular flap along with the EHB tendon are sutured to the plantar plate, taking care to protect the flexor hallucis longus (FHL) tendon and the plantar neurovascular bundles during suturing (**Fig. 3**A and B). The EHL tendon is then assessed to ensure no trauma has occurred during capsular flap creation or removal of dorsal osteophytes and its sheath is carefully repaired (**Fig. 4**A). ROM of the joint is then assessed, ensuring there is no block to dorsiflexion throughout the ROM arc (see **Fig. 4**B). The procedure is then completed with thorough irrigation, subcutaneous tissue closure, and skin closure with nylon suture.

Postoperative Protocol

Patients are weight-bearing as tolerated in a postoperative shoe for 4 weeks and are encouraged to begin immediate gentle passive ROM at home. Sutures are removed at 2 weeks, and radiographs are obtained at 6-week follow-up (**Fig. 5**).

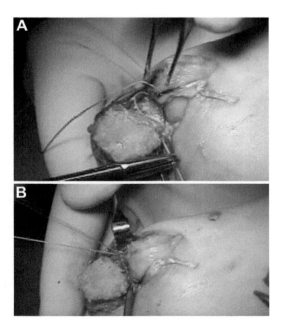

Fig. 3. (*A, B*) Using nonabsorbable suture, the previously raised capsular flap along is sutured to the plantar plate, taking care to protect the FHL tendon and the plantar neurovascular bundles during suturing.

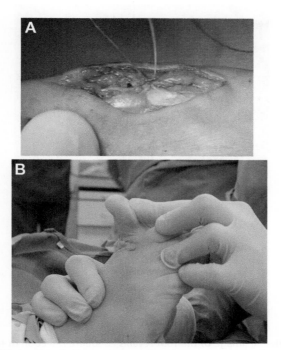

Fig. 4. (*A*) The EHL tendon is then assessed to ensure no trauma has occurred during capsular flap creation or removal of dorsal osteophytes and its sheath is carefully repaired. (*B*) ROM of the joint is then assessed, ensuring there is no block to dorsiflexion throughout the ROM arc.

Alternative Options

One may decide that the capsular tissue is inadequate. Alternative tissues have also been used. A dermal graft can be sutured to the dorsal metatarsal neck and then the dermal graft can either be sutured under the metatarsal head or it may be sutured under the head and then to the proximal phalanx. This will create a double layer of dermal graft between the bones (**Fig. 6**A–E). Another technique used is rolled tendon allograft as the interposition material.[1,2] These alternative techniques have not been studied as extensively as the capsular flap.

If capsular interposition arthroplasty fails, with continued pain, decreased ROM, and erosion into the proximal phalanx and metatarsal visible on radiographs, MTPJ arthrodesis with or without bone wedge allograft augmentation can be used as a salvage option.

LITERATURE REVIEW OF INTERPOSITIONAL ARTHROPLASTY

Interpositional arthroplasty and its variations have demonstrated adequate clinical outcomes and high patient satisfaction in the medium-term for the treatment of HR. The literature, however, contains substantial heterogeneity about surgical technique and reporting of specific outcome metrics. Moreover, there is insufficient evidence to provide a commentary regarding the durability of the procedure, with a paucity of series presenting long-term outcomes after these procedures. Thus, the purpose of this section is to provide an updated summary of the available literature concerning

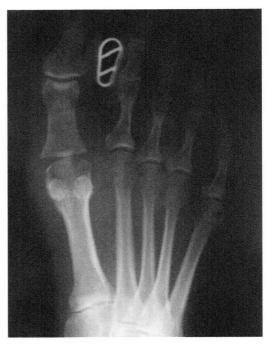

Fig. 5. Postoperative AP image of the foot reveals adequate resection of the proximal phalanx articular surface with interposed material.

the various forms of interpositional arthroplasty, with an emphasis on patient reported outcomes (PROs) and complication discussion.

Capsular Interpositional Arthroplasty

A majority of the studies to date regarding interpositional arthroplasty for HR have focused exclusively on capsular interpositional arthroplasty. Many studies, however, are limited by lack of long-term follow-up, thus precluding proper assessment of MTPJ arthrodesis conversion rates. Vulcano and colleagues published a series of 42 patients with mean follow-up of 11.2 years, the longest follow-up of the existing reports.[3] The visual analog scale, Foot Function Index, and Short Form 12 (SF-12) physical and mental scores all significantly improved from preoperative to final follow-up, indicating good functional outcomes in the long-term.[3] Similarly in another series, with mean follow-up of 9 years, patients who underwent a minimal resection capsular interpositional arthroplasty experienced significant improvements in their American Orthopedic Foot and Ankle Society-hallux metatarsal interphalangeal (AOFAS-HMI) score from preoperatively to postoperatively and 67% were able to tiptoe on their operative foot.[4] Significant improvements in AOFAS-HMI scores from preoperative to final follow-up have been found in studies with mid-term follow-up (mean 4.6–5.0 years), suggesting these functional improvements persist from mid-term to long-term.[5–10] Kennedy and colleagues[9] and Hahn and colleagues[11] included the SF-36 as part of their PRO measures and reported a mean of 96.3 and 72.9 after 3.2 years and 4.8 years, respectively.[9] The study conducted by Hahn and colleagues included patients with only grade IV HR, whereas Kennedy and colleagues included patients with grades II and III HR. This difference in severity as well as difference in follow-up may contribute to differences in final SF-36 scores.

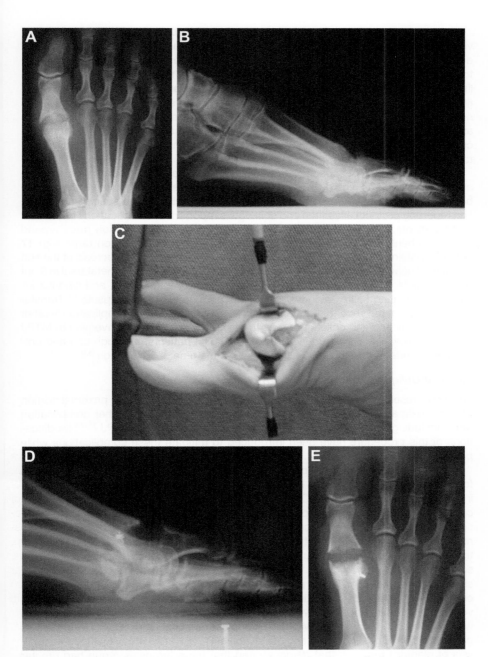

Fig. 6. (*A, B*) Preoperative AP and lateral radiographs reveal collapse of prior interpositional arthroplasty, with erosion into the proximal phalanx as well as the metatarsal. (*C*) Dissection is carried down to the level of the MTPJ, and the fibrotic tissue within the joint space is removed. The dermal allograft patch is placed over the metatarsal head and is held in place with 2 dorsal bone anchors. (*D, E*) Postoperative AP and lateral radiographs reveal maintained hallux alignment with restored joint space at the MTPJ.

In addition to functional improvements, capsular interpositional arthroplasty can provide improvements in ROM of the first MTPJ. Although studies with long-term follow-up did not assess ROM, several with mid-term follow-up demonstrated improvements in total ROM from preoperative to postoperative, ranging from 19.3° to 37° across the literature.[7–10,12] In addition, Clews and colleagues assessed dorsiflexion and plantarflexion separately and found significant increases in dorsiflexion postoperatively with no change in plantarflexion.[13] Commenting on changes in radiographic parameters after capsular interpositional arthroplasty for HR, Ozan and colleagues reported decreases in the mean hallux valgus angle (13.8°–10.2°) and increases in the intermetatarsal angle (10.5°–11.2°).[7]

Complication rates of capsular interpositional arthroplasty have been reported to be as low as 0% and as high as 82%.[5,14] The vast discrepancy across the literature can be attributed to substantial variation in described techniques and specific complication reporting protocol. Hamilton and colleagues reported no complications in a cohort of 14 patients, whereas other studies have shown low complication rates around 9%.[3,12] Schenk and colleagues had one of the highest complication rates with 17 out of 22 patients (77.2%) reporting complications. These included necrosis of the first metatarsal head in 9 out of 22 patients, metatarsalgia of the second metatarsal in 3 out of 22 patients, hypoesthesia of the big toe in 2 out of 22 patients, and singular instances of floating hallux, algodystrophy, and ossification of the capsule.[10] Transfer metatarsalgia of the second metatarsal was frequently cited as a complication in other studies.[4,7] Vulcano and colleagues was the only study to assess conversion to MTPJ fusion at a mean of 6.1 years in 4 out of 42 (9.5%) patients, although Lau and colleagues reported one patient awaiting fusion at the time of publication.[3,6]

Modified Oblique Keller Capsular Interpositional Arthroplasty

The Keller resection arthroplasty involves significant resection of the proximal portion of the proximal phalanx, which was hypothesized to result in higher complication rates, including very high rates of "floating toe" deformity at the MTPJ.[15,16] Modifications of this procedure have been introduced to mitigate these complications while preserving motion of the MTPJ.[5,17]

Sanhudo and colleagues reported outcomes of 25 cases with mean 3.2 years follow-up with grade III and IV HR who underwent modified oblique Keller capsular interpositional arthroplasty (MOKCIA) with cheilectomy and interposition of dorsal capsule and EHB.[18] The mean postoperative AOFAS score was 93.6 with a pain subscore of 36.4, functional subscore of 42.5, and alignment subscore of 14.7.[18] With regard to MTPJ mobility, 18 out of 25 (72%) of cases had mobility equal to or greater than 75° postoperatively.[18] Akgun and colleagues reported an identical mean AOFAS score in 13 cases with roughly 1 year less of follow-up.[19] Total active dorsiflexion ROM significantly improved in these patients from 6.5 to 51.9°.[19] Mackey and colleagues compared a cohort of 10 patients who underwent MOKCIA without cheilectomy versus 12 patients who underwent MTPJ arthrodesis and found that AOFAS scores were significantly higher in the MOKCIA group (89.6 vs 64.5, $P = .006$).[20] The MOKCIA group had 54° of passive ROM and 30° of active ROM.[20] This study included an analysis of plantar pressures that demonstrated that the arthrodesis group had greater pressure under the first metatarsal head but no difference in pressure under the second metatarsal head compared to the MOKCIA cohort.[20]

Of note, none of the studies discussed above reported any postoperative complications. However, in a systematic review conducted by Di Caprio and colleagues,[21] the overall complication rate following MOKCIA was 8.9% and rate of metatarsalgia was 1.1% in a group of 11 studies with long-term follow-up.[21] Further research with robust discussion of potential complications that can occur with MOKCIA will be required before the body of evidence can rival that which currently exists for traditional capsular interpositional arthroplasty. Moreover, further studies should move toward homogenous technique utilization for the procedures described as MOKCIA. Existing technique descriptions vary across the literature, precluding appropriate comparison with other motion-preserving options for HR.

Interpositional Arthroplasty with Other Soft Tissue Derivatives

In lieu of a capsular flap as interpositional material into the MTPJ space, techniques that use soft tissue alternatives have been developed. For instance, DelaCruz and colleagues published a series of 13 patients who underwent interpositional arthroplasty with meniscus allograft. At a mean follow-up of 16.5 months, the average AOFAS score improved from 52.5 to 90.0 with all patients showing improvement.[22] Mean dorsiflexion of the MTPJ improved from 15.8° to 47.77°.[22] No complications were recorded at short-term follow-up for this small cohort of patients. A higher complication rate was found in patients who underwent interpositional arthroplasty with tibialis anterior allograft rather than meniscus allograft. Thomas and colleagues presented 19 patients with mean follow-up of 1.3 years.[23] AOFAS scores improved from 68.5 to 74.1 postoperatively; however, 5 out of 19 (26%) patients required reoperations: 1 MTPJ, 1 bunionectomy, and 3 irrigation and debridements.[23] The large discrepancy between the complication rates reported by these 2 studies indicates the current limitations of the literature regarding interpositional arthroplasty for HR. It is highly unlikely that the choice of interposed allograft tissue (meniscus allograft vs tibialis anterior allograft) portends a substantially different complication rate but rather that approach and procedural techniques and follow-up and complication/outcome reporting methodologies account for this observed inconsistency.

Aynardi and colleagues present a larger cohort of patients who underwent interpositional arthroplasty with acellular dermal matrix with at least 2 years of follow-up and found the failure rate to be low at 3.6%.[24] Unfortunately, for other outcomes included in the study, patients who underwent interpositional arthroplasty with allograft were grouped with patients who underwent the procedure with autograft (capsule and EHB) with no subgroup analysis. Overall, 65.4% of the entire cohort (87 out of 133) reported excellent outcomes, and there were no significant differences in these PROs or rates of metatarsalgia between interposition types.[24] Furthermore, Carpenter and colleagues and Berlet and colleagues presented in isolation the short-term outcomes (mean 14 and 12.7 months) of patients who underwent interposition arthroplasty with acellular dermal matrix, with both studies reporting significantly increased postoperative AOFAS scores and no complications.[25,26]

An additional soft tissue option for interpositional arthroplasty is bovine pericardium collagen matrix. Of interest, bovine pericardium collagen matrix interpositional arthroplasty for HR is one of the few forms of interpositional arthroplasty that is backed by literature reporting long-term follow-up. Colo and colleagues presented 31 patients who all saw significant improvements in their AOFAS-HMI scores at final follow-up.[27] Mean follow-up for this cohort was 12.8 years. The rate of unsatisfying results was 16.1%, with 6.4% of patients with first ray shortening, 9.7% of patients with persistent metatarsal pain, and 1 case of complex regional pain syndrome.[27] No other reoperations or infections were reported. Further reports with long-term results are required to support the findings by Colo and colleagues but with satisfactory results at nearly 13-year average follow-up, bovine pericardium collagen matrix interpositional arthroplasty is an encouraging avenue for the motion-preserving treatment of HR.

Interpositional Arthroplasty with Gelfoam

Gelfoam-based interpositional arthroplasty has been proposed as a cheaper alternative to other joint replacement systems for the MTPJ, with several reports outlining similar functional and clinical outcomes. Heller and colleagues published a series of 31 patients with mean follow-up of 4.4 years and found that AOFAS-HMI scores improved from an average of 20 preoperatively to 74 at final follow-up.[28] These scores are similar to those found for other types of interpositional arthroplasty. The complication rate was found to be 3.2% with one patient that underwent arthrodesis after 6 months.[28] Long-term outcomes of Gelfoam-based interpositional arthroplasty techniques will be required before definitive statements regarding the efficacy of the procedure can be made.

SUMMARY

In summary, interpositional arthroplasty for the treatment of HR involves resection of the disease joint surface and placement of spacer material within the joint to preserve length at the MTPJ while still allowing for ROM. Regardless of specific subtype, interpositional arthroplasty has yielded good clinical and functional outcomes. That said, the majority of studies available in the literature have focused on capsular interpositional arthroplasty, leading to a larger subject pool and longer follow-up. Other forms of interpositional arthroplasty are less supported by long-term follow-up and large sample sizes. Moreover, there exists heterogeneity in the studies evaluating interpositional arthroplasty based on variation within outcome metrics and surgical techniques. Despite the limitations of the current data, interpositional arthroplasty seems to be a viable treatment option for HR with adequate functional and clinical outcomes that preserve ROM of the MTPJ.

CLINICS CARE POINTS

- The dorsomedial sensory cutaneous branch of the superficial peroneal nerve must be identified and protected carefully throughout any procedure approaching the hallux MTPJ.

- When raising a capsular flap for capsular interpositional arthroplasty from the proximal phalanx, care should be taken to ensure that as much capsular tissue as possible is lifted directly from the bone.

- A McGlamry elevator is an excellent tool to release the plantar plate and flexor hallucis brevis tendon from the plantar aspect of the proximal phalanx.

- The EHB can be mobilized into the joint space in addition to the capsular tissues to augment interpositional arthroplasty if more soft tissue material is required to maintain length of the first ray.

DISCLOSURE

The authors have no disclosures relevant to this article. Full disclosure information can be found on the American Academy of Orthopedic Surgery (AAOS) website.

SUPPLEMENTARY DATA

Supplementary data related to this article can be found online at https://doi.org/10.1016/j.fcl.2023.10.004.

REFERENCES

1. Watson TS, Panicco J, Parekh A. Allograft tendon interposition arthroplasty of the hallux metatarsophalangeal joint: a technique guide and literature review. Foot Ankle Int 2019;40(1):113–9.
2. Ferguson CM, Ellington JK. Operative technique: interposition arthroplasty and biological augmentation of hallux rigidus surgery. Foot Ankle Clin 2015;20(3):513–24.
3. Vulcano E, Chang AL, Solomon D, et al. Long-term follow-up of capsular interposition arthroplasty for hallux rigidus. Foot Ankle Int 2018;39(1):1–5.
4. Givissis PK, Symeonidis PD, Kitridis DM, et al. Minimal resection interposition arthroplasty of the first metatarsophalangeal joint. Foot 2017;32:1–7.
5. Hamilton WG, O'Malley MJ, Thompson FM, et al. Capsular interposition arthroplasty for severe hallux rigidus. Foot Ankle Int 1997;18(2):68–70.
6. Lau JT, Daniels TR. Outcomes following cheilectomy and interpositional arthroplasty in hallux rigidus. Foot Ankle Int 2001;22(6):462–70.
7. Fırat O, Osman Arslan B, Mehmet Ali FİLİZ ZK, et al. Interposition arthroplasty in the treatment of hallux rigidus. Acta Orthop Traumatol Turcica 2010;44(2):143–51.
8. Roukis TS, Landsman AS, Ringstrom JB, et al. Distally based capsule-periosteum interpositional arthroplasty for hallux rigidus: indications, operative technique, and short-term follow-up. J Am Podiatr Med Assoc 2003;93(5):349–66.
9. Kennedy JG, Chow FY, Dines J, et al. Outcomes after interposition arthroplasty for treatment of hallux rigidus. Clin Orthop Relat Res 2006;445:210–5.
10. Schenk S, Meizer R, Kramer R, et al. Resection arthroplasty with and without capsular interposition for treatment of severe hallux rigidus. Int Orthop 2009;33:145–50.
11. Hahn MP, Gerhardt N, Thordarson DB. Medial capsular interpositional arthroplasty for severe hallux rigidus. Foot Ankle Int 2009;30(6):494–9.
12. Hahn MP, Gerhardt N. Thordarson DB. Medial capsular interpositional arthroplasty for severe hallux rigidus. Foot Ankle Int 2009;30(6). https://doi.org/10.3113/FAI.2009.04.
13. Clews CN, Kingsford AC, Samaras DJ. Autogenous capsular interpositional arthroplasty surgery for painful hallux rigidus: assessing changes in range of motion and postoperative foot health. J Foot Ankle Surg 2015;54(1):29–36.
14. Butler JJ, Shimozono Y, Gianakos AL, et al. Interpositional arthroplasty in the treatment of hallux rigidus: a systematic review. J Foot Ankle Surg 2022;61(3):657–62.
15. Flamme H, Wülker N, Kuckerts K, et al. Follow-up results 17 years after resection arthroplasty of the great toe. Arch Orthop Trauma Surg 1998;117:457–60.
16. Majkowski RS, Galloway S. Excision arthroplasty for hallux valgus in the elderly: a comparison between the Keller and modified Mayo operations. Foot Ankle 1992;13(6):317–20.
17. Mroczek KJ, Miller SD. The modified oblique Keller procedure: a technique for dorsal approach interposition arthroplasty sparing the flexor tendons. Foot Ankle Int 2003;24(7):521–2.
18. Sanhudo JA, Gomes JE, Rodrigo MK. Surgical treatment of advanced hallux rigidus by interpositional arthroplasty. Foot Ankle Int 2011;32(4):400–6.
19. Akgun RC, Sahin O, Demirors H, et al. Analysis of modified oblique Keller procedure for severe hallux rigidus. Foot Ankle Int 2008;29(12):1203–8.

20. Mackey RB, Thomson AB, Kwon O, et al. The modified oblique keller capsular interpositional arthroplasty for hallux rigidus. J Bone Jt Surg Am Vol 2010;92(10): 1938.

21. Di Caprio F, Mosca M, Ceccarelli F, et al. Interposition arthroplasty in the treatment of end-stage hallux rigidus: a systematic review. Foot Ankle Spec 2021. https://doi.org/10.1177/19386400211053947. 19386400211053947.

22. DelaCruz EL, Johnson AR, Clair BL. First metatarsophalangeal joint interpositional arthroplasty using a meniscus allograft for the treatment of advanced hallux rigidus: surgical technique and short-term results. Foot Ankle Spec 2011;4(3): 157–64.

23. Thomas D, Thordarson D. Rolled tendon allograft interposition arthroplasty for salvage surgery of the hallux metatarsophalangeal joint. Foot Ankle Int 2018; 39(4):458–62.

24. Aynardi MC, Atwater L, Dein EJ, et al. Outcomes after interpositional arthroplasty of the first metatarsophalangeal joint. Foot Ankle Int 2017;38(5):514–8.

25. Berlet GC, Hyer CF, Lee TH, et al. Interpositional arthroplasty of the first MTP joint using a regenerative tissue matrix for the treatment of advanced hallux rigidus. Foot Ankle Int 2008;29(1):10–21.

26. Carpenter B, Duncan K, Ernst J, et al. Interposition ankle arthroplasty using acellular dermal matrix: a small series. J Foot Ankle Surg 2017;56(4):894–7.

27. Colò G, Fusini F, Alessio-Mazzola M, et al. Interposition arthroplasty with bovine collagenous membrane for hallux rigidus: A long-term results retrospective study. Foot Ankle Surg 2022;28(8):1473–8.

28. Heller E, Robinson D. Gelfoam first metatarsophalangeal replacement/interposition arthroplasty—a case series with functional outcomes. Foot 2011;21(3): 119–23.

Managing Hallux Rigidus in the Elite Athlete

Christopher D. Murawski, MD, Robert B. Anderson, MD*

KEYWORDS

- Hallux rigidus • Cheilectomy • First metatarsophalangeal joint • Athlete • Osteotomy
- Arthrodesis

KEY POINTS

- Hallux rigidus is the most common arthritic entity in the foot, as well as one of the most common foot and ankle entities for which active individuals seek advice and treatment due to pain and biomechanical implications.
- Surgical management can be considered where an athlete's athletic performance is limited.
- Outlining management strategies and return-to-play expectations with the athlete and his/her team are critical.

INTRODUCTION

Hallux rigidus is the most common arthritic entity in the foot,[1] as well as one of the most common foot and ankle entities for which active individuals seek advice and treatment due to pain and biomechanical implications. It is a localized, progressive degeneration of the hallux metatarsophalangeal (MP) joint, first described as "hallux flexus" by Davies-Colley.[2] In his initial description of this condition, he highlighted the plantar-flexed posture of the phalanx relative to the metatarsal head. The term "hallux rigidus" was subsequently coined by Cotterill[3] and remains commonly used today, along with the term "hallux limitus." Hallux limitus is typically regarded as a separate phenomenon whereby motion of the first MP joint is restricted without the presence of degenerative change.[4,5]

Although numerous theories have been proposed in terms of the etiology and pathophysiology of hallux rigidus, it has been generally considered to be a genetically predisposed condition given that most of the patients seem to endorse a family history.[6,7] Another theory is that of metatarsus elevatus, describing the dorsiflexed posture of the first ray and relationships with the foot and the consequent plantar-flexed posture of the hallux itself. This has been discussed by many authors, but

Foot & Ankle Institute, OrthoCarolina, 2001 Vail Avenue, Suite 200B, Charlotte, NC 28207, USA
* Corresponding author.
E-mail address: drrba1@gmail.com

Foot Ankle Clin N Am 29 (2024) 455–469
https://doi.org/10.1016/j.fcl.2023.12.004

foot.theclinics.com

the most current investigations have noted that this elevated posture of the first metatarsal improves after dorsal decompression of the hallux MP joint; therefore, it is likely a secondary rather than a primary observation.[6–10] Morphologic characteristics of a flat metatarsal head, as well as hallux valgus and metatarsus adductus, are likely to contribute to hallux rigidus.[5,6,11–13] Overuse etiologies and repetitive dorsiflexion forces may also lead to chondral injury and subsequent degeneration of the joint.[14] In this regard, prior reports have described osteochondral dissecans giving rise to a chronic hallux rigidus appearance.[15–17] Moreover, hallux rigidus of traumatic etiology, such as turf toe or hallux MP joint dislocation, can occur. In this article, the authors review the diagnosis as well as clinical considerations for managing hallux rigidus in the elite athlete.

CLINICAL GRADING

Clinical grading of hallux rigidus has been proposed by several authors in the past, this to assist in developing a treatment algorithm. The grading scales typically include mild to severe categories, which also may encompass grades ranging from 0 to 4 (with grade 0 being the mildest). Grading depends not only on the pathologic severity seen on radiographic evaluation but also on clinical parameters, including overall range of motion, mid-range pain and crepitus, the presence of sesamoid degeneration, and the size of the dorsal osteophyte of the first metatarsal head itself. Hattrup and Johnson created a radiographic classification scheme,[18] to which Easley and colleagues[19] added the prognostic importance of mid-range crepitus. This gave way to a more extensive grading scale by Coughlin and Shurnas[5], combining objective and subjective clinical data with radiographic findings.

CLINICAL PRESENTATION

The athlete who presents with hallux rigidus often notes symptoms with push-off activities, in addition to generalized hallux MP discomfort and swelling with vigorous activity.[6,20,21] In our experience, although the initial presentation may note bilateral evidence for hallux rigidus, it typically begins with unilateral symptoms.[22] The swelling and problematic dorsal bony prominence may interfere with athletic shoe wear, especially in soccer and football where athletes often prefer tightly fitting shoe wear. A paresthesia or dysesthesia to the dorsomedial aspect of the hallux may arise from external pressure on the cutaneous nerve coursing over the bony prominence.[23] Furthermore, transfer metatarsalgia may develop as a secondary biomechanical effect to the lack of hallux dorsiflexion.

Given the wide spectrum of presenting symptoms that can accompany a diagnosis of hallux rigidus, providing treatment recommendations to the athlete depends on what is problematic. As such, it is essential that the treating physician assess whether the pain is arising from extra-articular or intra-articular sources. Extra-articular sources of pain include a large bony prominence, bursitis, neuritis, or metatarsalgia, whereas intra-articular symptoms include pain and loss of motion due to the arthritic disease itself.

IMAGING

Imaging studies obtained in the evaluation of hallux rigidus include standing bilateral anteroposterior and lateral foot radiographs to allow for appropriate comparison of the symptomatic side to the contralateral side[22] (**Fig. 1**). Sesamoid views may be helpful to determine any osteophyte formation or advancing degenerative process.

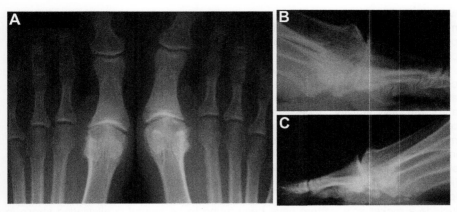

Fig. 1. Bilateral anteroposterior (*A*) and lateral (*B, C*) weight-bearing radiographs demonstrating bilateral hallux rigidus with dorsal osteophyte formation on both the first metatarsal and proximal phalanx, with congruent loss of joint space.

Fluoroscopic evaluation may assist in clearly delineating any restriction in motion to both plantarflexion and/or dorsiflexion. MRI can be helpful in quantifying the extent of joint degeneration and underlying subchondral edema that may assist with the discussion of surgical options and prognosis (**Fig. 2**).

CONSIDERATIONS FOR TREATMENT

Generally, treatment decisions also depend on the athlete's particular sport and position.[22] For example, a football lineman requires minimal hallux MP dorsiflexion to accomplish their performance needs; by comparison, a ballet performer or track athlete requires preservation of motion to remain competitive. As the improvement in overall motion of the affected joint is sought, it is essential that the physician outline the guarded prognosis to the athletic individual in that regard. To that end, the patient needs to understand that if the goal of surgical treatment is to provide increased motion through an already degenerative joint, it may degenerate more quickly and lead to

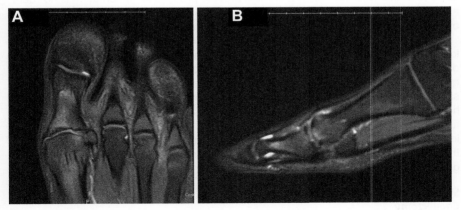

Fig. 2. Axial (*A*) and sagittal (*B*) T2 MRI sequences revealing hallux rigidus with dorsal osteophyte formation, as well as a large area of cartilage loss more centrally on the metatarsal head with corresponding subchondral edema, indicating more severe disease.

worsened symptoms and dysfunction over time. However, reasonable nonoperative modalities should be exhausted before considering surgical intervention and it is possible that approximately half of patients may find some degree of success with conservative management.[24]

There are number of nonoperative modalities that can be used for symptoms associated with hallux rigidus. The use of nonsteroidal anti-inflammatory medications or anti-inflammatory topical compounds may minimize some of the discomfort associated with daily activity. Shoe wear modifications that allow for accommodation of bony prominences and areas of swelling are recommended as well. Certain shoes may allow stretching of the upper toe box to provide more room for dorsal bony prominences. For athletes with dorsal impingement pain and who are able to tolerate a stiffer sole, the addition of a turf toe insert (eg, carbon fiber, aluminum) may be beneficial. These plates can be fitted to the distal half of the shoe to limit forefoot dorsiflexion while allowing preservation of midfoot and hindfoot motion. Running shoes that include a rocker sole pattern have been found to be helpful in alleviating stress in the hallux MP joint region. Orthotic devices can be prescribed to unload the hallux MP joint while providing relief of mechanical pressure on the sesamoid complex. One must keep in mind, however, that the introduction of an orthotic device will typically require an increase in shoe size to accommodate. Furthermore, injections to the hallux MP joint itself may be considered for both diagnostic and therapeutic purposes. Steroid and/or platelet-rich plasma (PRP) products may be used for this purpose and, in our experience, are best performed with fluoroscopic or ultrasound guidance and confirmation. In the case of steroid injections, symptomatic improvement is more likely in lower grades of disease.[25] Steroid injections should be given judiciously, as repeated injections may accelerate the degenerative process and create overlying soft tissue atrophy.[26] Hyaluronic acid injections in the management of hallux rigidus were not found to be superior in a single study comparing treatment to a steroid injection.[27] We are not aware of any studies assessing PRP injection in this setting.

Once pain and biomechanical issues limit an athlete's performance despite appropriate nonoperative modalities, he/she is likely to seek consultation for surgical intervention. There are several surgical options available in the management of hallux rigidus, but a lengthy preoperative discussion is mandatory with not only the athlete but also other parties involved in their sport and recovery process. It must be emphasized to all involved that this is a chronic arthritic process for which there is no "cure" and despite appropriate surgical techniques and rehabilitation, incomplete resolution of symptoms and dysfunction may occur, potentially preventing return to sport.

A preoperative evaluation necessitates a very thorough discussion of symptoms followed by a clinical examination that determines the origin of those symptoms and the degree of joint deterioration and motion restriction (**Fig. 3**). In that process, several questions will need to be answered[22]: (1) what is causing the problem? (2) is there dorsal irritation and impingement arising from a bony prominence over the metatarsal head with secondary shoe wear irritation? (3) is this a global arthritic process with painful motion even in the mid-range of the hallux MP joint? (4) are the sesamoids involved? and (5) what compensatory problems are developing? Answers to each of these questions will ultimately drive decision-making with respect to the particular surgical treatment performed.

SURGICAL MANAGEMENT STRATEGIES
Cheilectomy

This is likely the oldest and most commonly performed surgery in the management of hallux rigidus. This procedure is one in which the dorsal osteophyte of the first

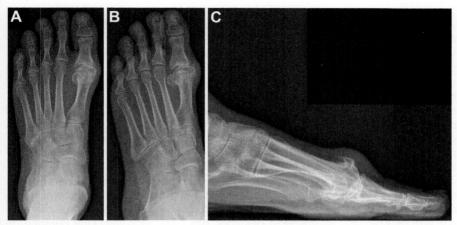

Fig. 3. Anteroposterior (*A*), oblique (*B*), and lateral (*C*) radiographs of the foot demonstrating hallux rigidus with large dorsal osteophyte, as well as a subluxed and incongruent first MP joint, yielding a difficult situation both for the athlete and treating surgeon.

metatarsal head is excised to an extent that allows for removal of impingement, thereby decompressing the dorsal bony prominence with the expectation of improved dorsiflexion through the joint. A cheilectomy may prolong the athletic life of an individual, but does not slow the rate of joint degeneration and while the dorsal osteophyte itself may not recur, progressive narrowing of the joint is expected following this procedure. A cheilectomy can be performed with any grade of hallux rigidus but is typically reserved for those with a dorsal bony prominence of the first metatarsal head and preservation of the joint space noted on a lateral radiograph. The best outcomes are typically found in those that do not exhibit pain or crepitus in the mid-range of motion, as well as pain in the sesamoid/metatarsal articulation. The attractiveness of a cheilectomy is inherent to the relatively simple procedure, affording a fairly rapid recovery and one in which "no bridges are burned."[28] Even with unsuccessful outcomes, a salvage procedure is still technically possible.

The technique described for accomplishing a cheilectomy was popularized by Mann and Clanton.[29] Their preference was performing the joint exposure through a dorsal longitudinal incision in which the dorsal 20% to 30% of the metatarsal head was removed along with the dorsal exostosis. Hamilton also recommended a plantar joint inspection with mobilization of the sesamoid complex, as these structures are often anchored by adhesions and could limit dorsiflexion even after adequate removal of the dorsal impinging osteophytes.[30] It has been generally agreed on that it is necessary to achieve a minimum of 70° to 80° of dorsiflexion intraoperatively, as much of this will be lost in the postoperative period as a result of scar formation. Easley and colleagues described a modification of the dorsal technique that used a medial incision to accomplish the cheilectomy but also allowed a more direct access to the sesamoid complex to include a plantar capsule release in an attempt to improve dorsiflexion.[19] Further, they recommended a two-cut technique to avoid excessive resection of the metatarsal head. The first cut with the saw included a removal of the dorsal exostosis flush with the dorsal diaphysis. The subsequent cut(s) removed eburnated bone on the dorsum of the metatarsal head along with the amount of articular surface necessary to achieve the desired dorsiflexion. This modification eliminated the risk of excessive head removal, which has the potential to jeopardize a later arthrodesis.

It is also reasonable to consider a joint-sparing cheilectomy in an athletic population with advanced radiographic disease but primarily dorsal symptoms when maintenance of motion is essential. Many authors have advocated a "radical" cheilectomy for those athletes with advanced stages of disease. Often referred to as the Valenti procedure,[31,32] an aggressive dorsal bone resection can be performed on both sides of the joint to allow for increased dorsiflexion, albeit with the risk of creating an unstable joint, as well as limiting future salvage opportunities. Colò and colleagues recently reported a retrospective series of 38 patients and 40 feet who underwent the Valenti procedure with a minimum 10-year follow-up and found significant improvements in a visual analog score, the Foot & Ankle Disability Index, as well as the American Orthopedic Foot and Ankle Society (AOFAS) Hallux Metatarsophalangeal-Interphalangeal Scale at the final follow-up.[33]

Recent advancements in minimally invasive surgical techniques and instrumentation have also yielded additional treatment options.[34–37] Specifically, accomplishing a dorsal decompression of the hallux MP joint through percutaneous portals and under arthroscopic and fluoroscopic guidance has been explored. One comparison study suggested that minimally invasive cheilectomy may carry a higher reoperation rate in comparison to open cheilectomy.[38] Future studies will be necessary to determine if this truly lessens the recovery process or improves the long-term outcome.

As mentioned previously, a standard open cheilectomy affords a relatively expedited postoperative course and return to activity. Weight-bearing is commenced immediately, typically in a rigid-soled sandal. The range of motion is initiated as pain permits, with aggressive icing to minimize swelling and inflammatory issues. The goal is to achieve a minimum of 40° of dorsiflexion, with patients being allowed to return to running and other athletic activities by 8 weeks.[22] Return to sport is based on discomfort and functional recovery.

There are number of articles discussing the results of cheilectomy. In the Mann and Clanton publication of 1988, 20 of 31 patients reported complete relief of pain and increased range of motion by an average of 20° in 31 feet.[29] However, this cohort was not composed of athletes. In fact, there are very few articles specifically outlining the success of cheilectomy in an elite athletic population. Mulier and colleagues reported on 20 athletes with 5-year follow-up and found it to be a reliable procedure in more mild grades of severity.[39] The general feeling among many authors, regardless of the patient population, has been that the procedure improves pain but not necessarily motion.

Phalangeal Osteotomy

A phalangeal osteotomy has been advocated as an adjuvant to a cheilectomy, typically when improved motion is not achieved through cheilectomy alone. This technique was first proposed in 1952 and early reports advocated for its use in adolescents with juvenile hallux rigidus in association with osteochondral lesions of the metatarsal head.[7] Moberg reported his case series in 1979 and is now the name commonly associated with the procedure.[40] The procedure involves a dorsal closing wedge osteotomy of the proximal third of the proximal phalanx and is based on the principal that the arc of motion of the hallux MP joint is translated to the plantar aspect of the metatarsal head, thereby increasing functional motion. Functionally, it creates pseudo-dorsiflexion, which as a result places less stress on the hallux with push-off. A prerequisite to the procedure is that there must be adequate plantar flexion of the joint preoperatively. An additional benefit to the procedure was described by Thomas and Smith,[41] noting that it provided dorsal joint space decompression, further relieving stress from the arthritic joint.

O'Malley and colleagues reported their results in managing advanced (Hattrup and Johnson grade III) hallux rigidus with cheilectomy and phalangeal extension osteotomy in 81 patients, of which 64 patients had complete 2-year follow-up.[42] At a mean follow-up of 4.3 years, 85.2% of patients were satisfied with the procedure. First MP joint motion improved significantly pre- to postoperatively, as did the mean AOFAS scores, which improved from a mean of 67.2 points preoperatively to 88.7 points postoperatively. Four patients subsequently requested first MP joint arthrodesis as a result of persistent symptoms.

Several hallux rigidus patients also have hallux valgus interphalangeus (**Fig. 4**). As a result, a modification to the Moberg procedure was published by Hunt and Anderson in the form of a biplanar closing wedge osteotomy of the proximal phalanx.[43] The technique included a cheilectomy, after which the dorsal medial incision was extended distally to expose the proximal phalanx. A Moberg-Akin osteotomy was created and internally fixed with a bicortical headless screw (**Fig. 5**). The investigators retrospectively reported the results of this procedure in 34 patients (35 feet) at an average follow-up of 22.5 months in which all osteotomies healed radiographically and 90% of patients achieved a good or excellent result. A single patient requested hardware removal. This cohort included athletes and is a procedure that represents a predictable surgical option for patients with combination hallux rigidus and hallux valgus interphalangeus.

The postoperative course for a phalangeal osteotomy procedure typically follows that of a cheilectomy, assuming rigid internal fixation has been achieved. This includes initiating passive dorsiflexion exercises at 1 to 2 weeks after surgery, with plantar flexion exercises typically delayed until 3 to 4 weeks postoperatively. Complications of a phalangeal osteotomy, whether a classic Moberg or biplanar technique, include that of nonunion or malunion. These complications can be avoided by "green sticking" the plantar cortex and creating gross instability.[22] Rigid internal fixation is mandatory in these cases. It is also recommended that intraoperative fluoroscopy be used to ensure that the osteotomy is made at the appropriate level, taking care to avoid any violation of the articular surface. The surgeon also needs to be cognizant of the flexor hallucis longus (FHL) and extensor hallucis longus (EHL) tendons and their locations such that iatrogenic injury can be avoided.

Metatarsal Osteotomies

In addition to phalangeal osteotomies, numerous techniques involving metatarsal osteotomies have been described, with mixed results. These techniques have included a sliding oblique metatarsal osteotomy,[44] a dorsiflexion closing wedge distal metatarsal osteotomy,[45] and an L-type shortening osteotomy,[46] among others. Saur and colleagues evaluated a retrospective cohort of 87 patients undergoing an oblique shortening distal metatarsal osteotomy and reported significant improvements in AOFAS score postoperatively for grades 1 to 3 hallux rigidus.[47] However, 15 patients

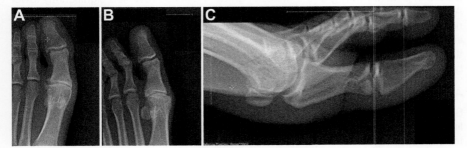

Fig. 4. Anteroposterior (A), oblique (B), and lateral (C) radiographs of the first ray revealing hallux rigidus with an interphalangeus deformity of the proximal phalanx.

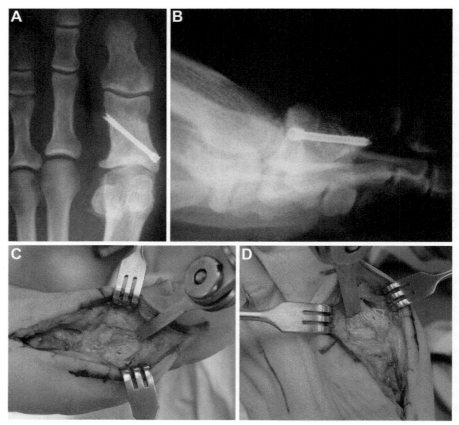

Fig. 5. Anteroposterior (*A*) and lateral (*B*) radiographs of the hallux status post dorsal cheilectomy and a Moberg-Akin osteotomy of the proximal phalanx fixed with a single headless screw. Intraoperative images demonstrate the oblique biplanar nature of the osteotomy (*C, D*).

reported symptoms of transfer metatarsalgia at the 6-month follow-up. Separately, Cho and colleagues reported 42 cases in 39 patients of a distal metatarsal dorsiflexion osteotomy for grades 3 to 4 hallux rigidus.[45] Although predictable pain relief was reported in patients with grade 3 disease, grade 4 disease revealed significantly lower AOFAS scores and a higher rate of reoperation for persistent symptoms. In the experience of the current authors, concerns associated with metatarsal osteotomies include malunion with transfer metatarsalgia or sesamoiditis, arthrofibrosis (including the sesamoid complex) with stiffness, and cock-up deformity of the hallux and should be used with caution.

Arthroplasty

Salvage options for those who fail cheilectomy, with or without an osteotomy, are quite limited in the athletic population. Although arthrodesis provides a permanent solution to advanced degeneration, it is not feasible in the individual who requires maintenance of motion to continue at a competitive level in sport-related activities. This is particularly true for any running athlete or dancer. In this regard, arthroplasty techniques have been described. Implant arthroplasty has not shown success in the active individual due to loosening and failure of the implants leading to a significant segmental bony defect.[48–50] The use of a Hydrogel spacer, while met with initial intrigue,[51–53] led to failure with pain, subsidence, and stiffness.[54–56] Therefore, resection/interposition arthroplasty techniques have been described for those requiring maintenance of motion.

The oldest of these techniques is the Keller resection arthroplasty, which is reserved for older individuals due to the secondary issues of hallux instability, malalignment, and lack of push-off. Hamilton devised a modification of this procedure, which entailed capsular interposition in conjunction with a less aggressive resection of the proximal phalanx.[57,58] However, the extensor hallucis brevis (EHB) tendon, extensor hood and dorsal capsule were often found to be insufficient in providing adequate soft tissue interposition. Conical resection on both sides of the joint followed by insertion of a hamstring allograft rolled into an "anchovy" was described by Coughlin in a small case series.[59] We have found success using this on several athletes in the short term, but the large bone defect created was of concern for later salvage. This technique, however, is an option to consider when one fails a bipolar implant arthroplasty and wishes to avoid an arthrodesis. Our preference in these resection options is the technique described by Berlet and colleagues, which uses "parachute" dermal allograft coverage of the metatarsal head in conjunction with a Valenti resection on the base of the proximal phalanx that preserves the plantar plate.[60] We have found this technique to provide not only good pain relief but also maintain good push-off strength and FHL function (**Fig. 6**).

The postoperative course after a soft tissue interposition arthroplasty performed in isolation is relatively simple. We allow for immediate weight-bearing in a hard-sole sandal and initiation of gentle range of motion at 2 weeks. Hallux alignment is maintained with a removal splint apparatus. Running commences at 8 weeks postsurgically with emphasis on FHL strengthening. The anticipated return to sport averages 4 months. Complications of a soft-tissue arthroplasty include, first and foremost, persistent pain and lack of functional motion. The lack of push-off power and instability is also problematic. Some patients will develop a gradual valgus and/or dorsiflexion drift of the hallux, making shoewear difficult. The only salvage for these issues is an arthrodesis.

Arthrodesis

When even salvage procedures such as interposition arthroplasty fail to provide relief for improved motion, arthrodesis may be necessary. If it is to be performed, the toe tip

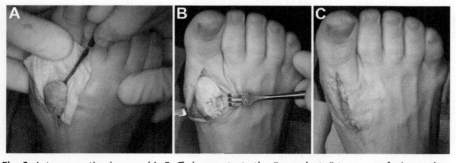

Fig. 6. Intraoperative images (*A, B, C*) demonstrate the "parachute" type resurfacing arthroplasty procedure in which a dermal allograft is used to cover the metatarsal head as a salvage procedure to avoid arthrodesis.

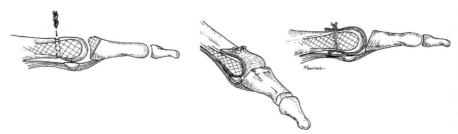

Fig. 7. The interpositional arthroplasty technique with a modified Keller resection of the proximal phalanx and subsequent placement and fixation of dermal allograft to the metatarsal head. (*Reproduced from* Berlet GC, Hyer CF, Lee TH, Philbin TM, Hartman JF, Wright ML. Interpositional arthroplasty of the first MTP joint using a regenerative tissue matrix for the treatment of advanced hallux rigidus. Foot Ankle Int. 2008 Jan;29(1):10-21.)

should be at least 10 mm off the ground in a "running" athletic population.[22] Failure to meet this requirement will place significant stress on the distal hallux and plantar aspect of the interphalangeal (IP) joint; this will lead to plantar callus and pain, as well as the potential for instability and dorsiflexion of the hallux IP joint itself. A slight shortening of the hallux through the arthrodesis may also be beneficial in the running athlete, as it further lessens the potential for the patient having to "vault" over the hallux during running activity.

Da Cunha and colleagues assessed sports and physical activities in a younger patient population between the ages of 18 and 55 years who underwent first MP joint fusion with a minimum 2-year follow-up.[61] In their study, 50 patients with a mean follow-up of 5.1 years reported participating in a range of high- and low-impact sporting activities, with 96% of patients being satisfied with the procedure and their ability to resume physical activities. The median time to return to physical activity was 6 to 9 months, whereas the median time to reach maximal physical activity levels was 9 to 12 months. In fact, no single patient reported that they had discontinued their desired physical activities pre- to postoperatively, but patients began participating in 21 new physical activities. Postoperative patient-specific physical activities were rated as improved in difficulty in 27.4%, the same difficulty in 51.2% and more difficult in 21.4% of patients. The results of this study suggest that in younger and active patients who require definitive management with first MP joint fusion, the majority will return to their desired athletic activities with either the same or an improved level of difficulty.

Osteochondral Lesions of the First Metatarsophalangeal Joint

Osteochondral lesions of the metatarsal head are a unique pathology frequently associated with a traumatic episode that can present in isolation, frequently with pain and/

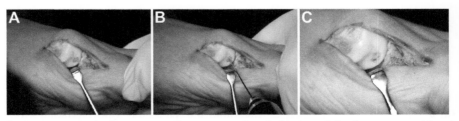

Fig. 8. Intraoperative images revealing an osteochondral lesion of the first metatarsal head (*A*) with subsequent drilling of the lesion (*B, C*).

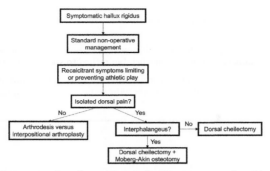

Fig. 9. Flowchart demonstrating the senior author's treatment algorithm in elite/competitive athletes.

or mechanical MP joint symptoms, or in combination with symptoms of hallux rigidus.[62–64] Although radiographs are often normal, they should be carefully assessed for lucency in the central metatarsal head region. Differentiating the source of pain in combination pathologies can be challenging. An MRI is useful when pain and dysfunction persist, as it may highlight localized edema in the central metatarsal head. When conservative therapies are exhausted, surgical management may be necessary. Ter Laak Bolk and colleagues reported a small case series of nine patients with focal osteochondral lesions of the first MP joint, of which eight patients were located on the first MP head and treated with first MP joint arthroscopy and bone marrow stimulation.[65] Seven of these patients were involved with competitive or elite levels of sport, of which six returned to sport at a median of 4 months, including five at the preoperative level. Other small case reports describe further treatment strategies, including osteochondral autograft transplant.[66–68] Our preference has been an open exploration with management of the lesion consisting of excision of the loose chondral flap, microfracture, cartilage allograft implantation when size permits, and a cheilectomy, when needed (**Fig. 7**). Further work is required in this realm of an uncommon pathology.

SUMMARY

Hallux rigidus can present a difficult problem to both competitive and elite athletic populations. When reasonable conservative measures fail to allow the athlete to compete at their desired level, surgical intervention is often performed (**Figs. 8 and 9**). In the experience of the senior author, a joint-sparing cheilectomy, in addition to a dorsal closing wedge or biplanar closing wedge osteotomy of the proximal phalanx, when necessary, can provide a predictable return to sport at the most elite levels. Arthroplasty or arthrodesis techniques can be used for persistent symptoms or progressive disease, albeit with less predictable outcomes with respect to returning to sports. Preoperative discussion with the athlete and his/her team is essential to outline management and return to play expectations.

CLINICS CARE POINTS

- Hallux rigidus can present a difficult problem to both competitive and elite athletic populations.

- Discussion and education of the athlete and his/her team is essential to outline management and return to play expectations.
- A joint-sparing cheilectomy ± a dorsal closing wedge or biplanar closing wedge osteotomy of the proximal phalanx can provide a predictable return to sport at the most elite levels.
- Arthroplasty or arthrodesis techniques can be used for persistent symptoms or progressive disease, albeit with less predictable outcomes with respect to returning to high-level sport activities.

DISCLOSURE

C.D. Murawski has none relevant to this article; American Orthopedic Foot and Ankle Society–Research Committee. R.B. Anderson has none relevant to this article; Consultant/Royalties from Stryker; Consultant for Arthrex, Enovis, BioTissue, Artelon, NuVasive, Osteoremedies.

REFERENCES

1. van Saase JL, van Romunde LK, Cats A, et al. Epidemiology of osteoarthritis: zoetermeer survey. comparison of radiological osteoarthritis in a dutch population with that in 10 other populations. Ann Rheum Dis 1989;48(4):271–80.
2. Davies-Colley M. Contraction of the metatarsophalangeal joint of the great toe. Br Med J 1887;1:728.
3. Cotterill JM. Condition of the stiff great toe in adolescents. Br Med J 1887; 1(1378):1158.
4. Viehöfer AF, Vich M, Wirth SH, et al. The role of plantar fascia tightness in hallux limitus: a biomechanical analysis. J Foot Ankle Surg 2019;58(3):465–9.
5. Coughlin MJ, Shurnas PS. Hallux rigidus. grading and long-term results of operative treatment. J Bone Joint Surg Am 2003;85-A(11):2072–88.
6. Anderson MR, Ho BS, Baumhauer JF. Republication of "current concepts review: hallux rigidus". Foot Ankle Orthop 2023;8(3). 24730114231188123.
7. Bonney G, Macnab I. Hallux valgus and hallux rigidus; a critical survey of operative results. J Bone Joint Surg Br 1952;34-B(3):366–85.
8. Horton GA, Park YW, Myerson MS. Role of metatarsus primus elevatus in the pathogenesis of hallux rigidus. Foot Ankle Int 1999;20(12):777–80.
9. Jack EA. The aetiology of hallux rigidus. Br J Surg 1940;27:492–7.
10. Lambrinudi C. Metatarsus primus elevates. Proc Roy Soc Med 1938;31(11):1273.
11. Coughlin MJ, Shurnas PS. Hallux rigidus: demograpics, etiology, and radiographic assessment. Foot Ankle Int 2003;24(10):731–43.
12. D'Arcangelo PR, Landorf KB, Munteanu SE, et al. Radiographic correlates of hallux valgus severity in older people. J Foot Ankle Res 2010;3:20.
13. DuVries HL. DuVries' surgery of the foot. St. Louis: Mosby; 1959.
14. McMaster MJ. The pathogenesis of hallux rigidus. J Bone Joint Surg Br 1978; 60(1):82–7.
15. Kelikian H. Hallux valgus: allied deformities of the forefoot and metatarsalgia. Philadelphis: WB Saunders; 1965.
16. Goodfellow J. Aetiology of hallux rigidus. Proc Roy Soc Med 1966;59(9):821–4.
17. Kessel L, Bonney G. Hallux rigidus in the adolescent. J Bone Joint Surg Br 1958; 40-B(4):669–73.
18. Hattrup SJ, Johnson KA. Hallux rigidus: a review. Adv Orthop Surg 1986;9: 259–63.

19. Easley ME, Davis WH, Anderson RB. Intermediate to long-term follow-up of medial-approach dorsal cheilectomy for hallux rigidus. Foot Ankle Int 1999; 20(3):147–52.
20. Heller WA, Brage ME. The effects of cheilectomy on dorsi- flexion of the first meta-tarsophalangeal joint. Foot Ankle Int 1997;18(12):803–8.
21. Shereff MJ, Bejjani FJ, Kummer FJ. Kinematics of the first metatarsophalangeal joint. J Bone Joint Surg Am 1986;68(3):392–8.
22. Anderson RB, Shawen SB. Great-toe disorders. In: Porter DA, Schon LC, editors. Baxter's the foot and ankle in sport. 2nd edition. Philadelphia, PA: Elsevier Health Sciences; 2007. p. 411–33.
23. Keiserman LS, Sammarco VJ, Sammarco GJ. Surgical treatment of the hallux rigidus. Foot Ankle Clin 2005;10(1):75–96.
24. Grady JF, Axe TM, Zager EJ, et al. A retrospective analysis of 772 patients with hallux limitus. J Am Podiatr Med Assoc 2002;92(2):102–8.
25. Solan MC, Calder JD, Bendall SP. Manipulation and injection for hallux rigidus. Is it worthwhile? J Bone Joint Surg Br 2001;83(5):706–8.
26. Thompson FL. Surgery of the foot and ankle. 6th edition. St. Louis: Mosby; 1993.
27. Pons M, Alvarez F, Solana J, et al. Sodium hyaluronate in the treatment of hallux rigidus. a single-blind, randomized study. Foot Ankle Int 2007;28(1):38–42.
28. Rajan L, Kim J, An T, et al. Effect of prior cheilectomy on outcomes of first meta-tarsophalangeal joint fusion for treatment of hallux rigidus. Foot Ankle Orthop 2022;7(3). 24730114221119740.
29. Mann RA, Clanton TO. Hallux rigidus: treatment by cheilectomy. J Bone Joint Surg Am 1988;70(3):400–6.
30. Hamilton WG. Foot and ankle injuries in dancers. Clin Sports Med 1988;7(1): 143–73.
31. Kurtz DH, Harrill JC, Kaczander BI, et al. The Valenti procedure for hallux limitus: a long-term follow-up and analysis. J Foot Ankle Surg 1999;38(2):123–30.
32. Saxena A. The Valenti procedure for hallux limitus/rigidus. J Foot Ankle Surg 1995;34(5):485–8, discussion 511.
33. Colò G, Alessio-Mazzola M, Dagnino G, et al. Long-term results of surgical treatment of valenti procedures for hallux rigidus: a minimum ten-year follow-up retrospective study. J Foot Ankle Surg 2019;58(2):291–4.
34. Hunt KJ. Hallux metatarsophalangeal (MTP) joint arthros- copy for hallux rigidus. Foot Ankle Int 2015;36(1):113–9.
35. Iqbal MJ, Chana GS. Arthroscopic cheilectomy for hallux rigidus. Arthroscopy 1998;14(3):307–10.
36. Walter R, Perera A. Open, arthroscopic, and percutaneous cheilectomy for hallux rigidus. Foot Ankle Clin 2015;20:421–31.
37. Kaplan DJ, Chen JS, Colasanti CA, et al. Needle arthroscopy cheilectomy for hallux rigidus in the office setting. Arthrosc Tech 2022;11(3):e385–90.
38. Stevens R, Bursnall M, Chadwick C, et al. Comparison of complication and reoperation rates for minimally invasive versus open cheilectomy of the first metatar-sophalangeal joint. Foot Ankle Int 2020;41(1):31–6.
39. Mulier T, Steenwerckx A, Thienpont E, et al. Results after cheilectomy in athletes with hallux rigidus. Foot Ankle Int 1999 Apr;20(4):232–7.
40. Moberg E. A simple operation for hallux rigidus. Clin Orthop Relat Res 1979;(142):55–6.
41. Thomas PJ, Smith RW. Proximal phalanx osteotomy for the surgical treatment of hallux rigidus. Foot Ankle Int 1999;20(1):3–12.

42. O'Malley MJ, Basran HS, Gu Y, et al. Treatment of advanced stages of hallux rigidus with cheilectomy and phalangeal osteotomy. J Bone Joint Surg Am 2013; 95(7):606–10.
43. Hunt KJ, Anderson RB. Biplanar proximal phalanx closing wedge osteotomy for hallux rigidus. Foot Ankle Int 2012;33(12):1043–50.
44. Nakajima K. Sliding oblique metatarsal osteotomy fixated with k-wires without cheilectomy for all grades of hallux rigidus: a case series of 76 patients. Foot Ankle Orthop 2022;7(4). 24730114221144048.
45. Cho BK, Park KJ, Park JK, et al. Outcomes of the distal metatarsal dorsiflexion osteotomy for advanced hallux rigidus. Foot Ankle Int 2017;38(5):541–50.
46. Ceccarini P, Ceccarini A, Rinonapoli G, et al. Outcome of distal first metatarsal osteotomy shortening in hallux rigidus grades II and III. Foot Ankle Int 2015; 36(12):1469–74.
47. Saur M, Lucas Y, Hernandes J, et al. Average 4-year outcomes of distal oblique first metatarsal osteotomy for stage 1 to 3 hallux rigidus. Foot Ankle Int 2022; 43(4):463–73.
48. Cracchiolo A 3rd, Weltmer JB Jr, Lian G, et al. Arthroplasty of the first metatarsophalangeal joint with a double-stem silicone implant. Results in patients who have degenerative joint disease failure of previous operations, or rheumatoid arthritis. J Bone Joint Surg Am 1992;74(4):552–63.
49. Gibson JN, Thomson CE. Arthrodesis or total replacement arthroplasty for hallux rigidus: a randomized controlled trial. Foot Ankle Int 2005;26(9):680–90.
50. Raikin SM, Ahmad J, Pour AE, et al. Comparison of arthrodesis and metallic hemiarthroplasty of the hallux metatarsophalangeal joint. J Bone Joint Surg Am 2007; 89(9):1979–85.
51. Baumhauer JF, Singh D, Glazebrook M, et al, for and on behalf of the CARTIVA Motion Study Group. Prospective, randomized, multi-centered clinical trial assessing safety and efficacy of a synthetic cartilage implant versus first metatarsophalangeal arthrodesis in advanced hallux rigidus. Foot Ankle Int 2016;37(5): 457–69.
52. Daniels TR, Younger AS, Penner MJ, et al. Midterm outcomes of polyvinyl alcohol hydrogel hemiarthroplasty of the first metatarsophalangeal joint in advanced hallux rigidus. Foot Ankle Int 2017;38(3):243–7.
53. Goldberg A, Singh D, Glazebrook M, et al, Cartiva MOTION Study Group. Association between patient factors and outcome of synthetic cartilage implant hemiarthroplasty vs first metatarsophalangeal joint arthrodesis in advanced hallux rigidus. Foot Ankle Int 2017;38(11):1199–206.
54. Shimozono Y, Hurley ET, Kennedy JG. Early failures of polyvinyl alcohol hydrogel implant for the treatment of hallux rigidus. Foot Ankle Int 2021;42(3):340–6.
55. Cassinelli SJ, Chen S, Charlton TP, et al. Early outcomes and complications of synthetic cartilage implant for treatment of hallux rigidus in the United States. Foot Ankle Int 2019;40(10):1140–8.
56. Akoh CC, Chen J, Kadakia R, et al. Adverse events involving hallux metatarsophalangeal joint implants: analysis of the United States food and drug administration data from 2010 to 2018. Foot Ankle Surg 2021;27(4):381–8.
57. Hamilton WG, O'Malley MJ, Thompson FM, et al. Capsular interposition arthroplasty for severe hallux rigidus. Foot Ankle Int 1997;18(2):68–70.
58. Hamilton WG, Hubbard CE. Hallux rigidus. excisional arthroplasty. Foot Ankle Clin 2000;5(3):663–71.
59. Coughlin MJ, Shurnas PJ. Soft-tissue arthroplasty for hallux rigidus. Foot Ankle Int 2003;24(9):661–72.

60. Berlet GC, Hyer CF, Lee TH, et al. Interpositional arthroplasty of the first MTP joint using a regenerative tissue matrix for the treatment of advanced hallux rigidus. Foot Ankle Int 2008;29(1):10–21.
61. Da Cunha RJ, MacMahon A, Jones MT, et al. Return to sports and physical activities after first metatarsophalangeal joint arthrodesis in young patients. Foot Ankle Int 2019;40(7):745–52.
62. Waldrop NE 3rd. Assessment and treatment of sports injuries to the first metatarsophalangeal joint. Foot Ankle Clin 2021;26(1):1–12.
63. Coker TP, Arnold JA, Weber DL. Traumatic lesions of the metatarsophalangeal joint of the great toe in athletes. Am J Sports Med 1978;6(6):326–34.
64. Street CC, Shereff MJ. Traumatic osteochondral defect of the first metatarsal head: a case report. Am J Orthop (Belle Mead NJ) 1999;28(10):584–6.
65. Ter Laak Bolk CS, Rikken QGH, Dahmen J, et al. Back in action: high return to pre-injury level of sports after arthroscopic bone marrow stimulation for osteochondral lesions of the first metatarsophalangeal (MTP-1) joint. Cartilage 2023; 21. 19476035231200332.
66. Kim YS, Park EH, Lee HJ, et al. Clinical comparison of the osteochondral autograft transfer system and subchondral drilling in osteochondral defects of the first metatarsal head. Am J Sports Med 2012;40(8):1824–33.
67. Van Dyke B, Berlet GC, Daigre JL, et al. First metatarsal head osteochondral defect treatment with particulated juvenile cartilage allograft transplantation: a case series. Foot Ankle Int 2018;39(2):236–41.
68. Artioli E, Mazzotti A, Zielli SO, et al. Surgical management of osteochondral lesions of the first metatarsal head: a systematic review. Foot Ankle Surg 2023; 29(5):387–92.

Minimally Invasive Cheilectomy for Hallux Rigidus

Amanda N. Fletcher, MD, MSc[a],[*],[1], Vandan Patel, MD[b],
Rebecca Cerrato, MD[c]

KEYWORDS

- Minimally invasive surgery • Hallux rigidus • Cheilectomy

KEY POINTS

- Hallux metatarsophalangeal joint cheilectomy is a joint-sparing technique that involves resection of the dorsal metatarsal head osteophytes; this may be achieved through minimally invasive and arthroscopic techniques.
- General indications for minimally invasive surgery (MIS) cheilectomy are mild-to-moderate hallux rigidus (Grades I–II) with symptomatic dorsal osteophytes causing dorsal impingement and/or shoe wear irritation in those who have failed extensive nonoperative management.
- The literature confirms equivalent outcomes to open cheilectomy; however, it is somewhat inconsistent regarding superiority.
- The theoretic benefits of MIS cheilectomy include better cosmesis, reduced wound complications, less soft tissue disruption, and faster recovery.

INTRODUCTION/HISTORY/DEFINITIONS/BACKGROUND

Hallux rigidus is a common degenerative condition of the first metatarsophalangeal (MTP) joint, characterized by cartilage loss, joint space narrowing, marginal osteophyte formation, loss of motion, and pain. Hallux rigidus is most common in patients aged older than 40 years with a 2:1 female-to-male predominance.[1,2] Classically, dorsal osteophytes involving both the metatarsal and proximal phalanx result in dorsal impingement with MTP joint dorsiflexion. Patients may also develop medial osteophytes and can present for evaluation of a painful bunion.[2] Dorsal impingement typically manifests as pain with push off during ambulation and shoe wear irritation from

[a] OrthoCarolina, 2001 Vail Avenue, Suite 200B, Charlotte, NC 28207-1222, USA; [b] Department of Orthopaedic Surgery, University of Michigan, 2098 S Main Street, Ann Arbor, MI 48103, USA; [c] Mercy Medical Center, Baltimore, The Institute for Foot and Ankle Reconstruction, 301 St Paul Place, Institute for Foot and Ankle Reconstruction At Mercy, Baltimore, MD 21202, USA
[1] Present address: 915 S Wolfe Street, Apt# 136, Baltimore, MD, 21231.
* Corresponding author. 2001 Vail Avenue, Suite 200B, Charlotte, NC 28207-1222.
E-mail address: Amanda.fletcher@orthocarolina.org

Foot Ankle Clin N Am 29 (2024) 471–484
https://doi.org/10.1016/j.fcl.2024.01.003
1083-7515/24/© 2024 Elsevier Inc. All rights reserved.

direct pressure on the prominent osteophytes. Patients may also present with abnormal gait mechanics with lateral boarder overload or even peroneal tendonitis in an attempt to minimize pain at the first MTP joint.[3]

There have been a couple of different grading systems for hallux rigidus to help characterize the extent of disease. The Hattrup-Johnson classification is a simple radiographic grading system. Grade I is mild-to-moderate osteophyte formation with good joint space preservation, Grade II is moderate osteophyte formation with joint space narrowing and subchondral sclerosis, and Grade III is marked osteophyte formation and loss of visible joint space with or without subchondral cyst formation.[4] The Coughlin-Shurnas classification was described in 2003 and combines clinical and radiographic findings to grade the extent of disease.[5] Although these grading systems can help guide treatment options, patient-specific factors including age, sex, bone quality, lifestyle, and goals should weigh heavily on the decision.

Initial management consists of various nonoperative modalities including activity modification, shoe wear modification, and anti-inflammatories. Shoe wear modifications include rigid-soled shoes, rigid inserts with Morton's extension limiting hallux MTP dorsiflexion, wider toe boxes, and deeper toe boxes to limit dorsal irritation.[1] Anti-inflammatories and corticosteroid injections may also provide symptomatic relief. Following failure of nonoperative management and persistent functional limitations, surgical options range from joint-sparing procedures including cheilectomy and osteotomies to joint sacrificing procedures including arthroplasty and arthrodesis.[6]

Cheilectomy is a joint-sparing technique that involves resection of the dorsal metatarsal head osteophytes and some degree of the metatarsal head. Cheilectomy is indicated in early disease stages where symptoms are predominantly related to the presence of dorsal osteophytes and dorsal impingement with the preservation of joint space and motion. The procedure decreases dorsal impingement pain, shoe wear irritation, dorsiflexion of the hallux MTP, and gait function because it increases the peak ankle push-off power in the sagittal plane.[7] Appropriate preoperative counseling and expectation setting is imperative, specifically the primary goal of pain relief rather than motion gain. Additionally, the procedure does not eliminate the ongoing degenerative process within the joint, which may require repeat surgery in the future. A benefit of cheilectomy is that it permits later use of any other procedure. In rare situations, a patient may present with advanced disease with only complaints of the dorsal prominence hurting in shoe wear. Despite the advanced degenerative stage, these patients can benefit from a cheilectomy procedure.

With the advent and popularization of minimally invasive surgery (MIS), cheilectomy is now possible through poke-hole incisions. The development of procedure-specific equipment and instruments has advanced MIS techniques. MIS procedures have the theoretic benefits of smaller incisions, improved cosmesis, less soft tissue trauma and scarring, and faster recovery compared to their open counterparts. Small joint arthroscopy has also been introduced to supplement MIS procedures with direct visualization and examination of the joints.[8]

Indications and Contraindications

General indications for MIS cheilectomy are mild-to-moderate hallux rigidus with symptomatic dorsal osteophytes causing dorsal impingement and/or shoe wear irritation in those who have failed extensive nonoperative management.[9] Patients with greater than 6 months of pain, dorsal-based symptoms, pain at extremes of motion, greater than 50% joint space preservation, radiographic dorsal osteophyte, and minimal sagittal or axial plane deformity of the metatarsal are indicated. Experience with MIS and small joint arthroscopic instruments and techniques is a relative indication.

Contraindications include advanced arthritis with a positive grind test, greater than 50% joint space narrowing, midrange pain with passive MTP motion (Coughlin-Shurnas grade IV),[5] plantar or sesamoid pain, night or rest pain, lack of dorsal osteophyte, infection or compromised soft tissue, and joint malalignment necessitating corrective osteotomies.[9-12] Although the literature describes success with up to grade III hallux rigidus, we recommend MIS cheilectomy in patients with grades I to II hallux rigidus with greater than 50% joint space preservation and dorsal osteophytes causing impingement pain at terminal dorsiflexion. Each patient should be evaluated individually with care to understand their symptoms, lifestyle, functional limitations, and goals of care.

Preoperative Planning

A thorough and systematic history and physical should be performed. Hallux MTP joint range of motion should be measured and documented. This can be measured using the axis of the proximal phalanx relative to the plantar surface of the foot or relative to the axis of the first metatarsal. The interphalangeal joint must be held in neutral to avoid overestimating motion. Careful examination of pain with passive motion of the MTP joint must be documented. Pain at terminal dorsiflexion indicates dorsal impingement, whereas pain at mid-arc motion and a positive MTP grind test indicate advanced degenerative changes. The soft tissue envelope and skin should be examined for signs of infection or compromise. Skin hypertrophy or erythema can also indicate shoe wear irritation at the dorsomedial prominence.

Weight-bearing radiographs should include anteroposterior (AP), oblique, and lateral views of the affected foot. The AP view can be used to evaluate the condition of the joint space, marginal osteophytes, alignment of the first ray, and condition of the surrounding joints. The oblique view can show additional osteophytes and joint space narrowing. The lateral view demonstrates the size and extent of the dorsal osteophytes on both the metatarsal head and base of the proximal phalanx as well as further characterizes the joint space narrowing. Advanced imaging is rarely indicated but can be helpful in assessing suspected intra-articular pathology or for atypical symptomatology.

Surgical Technique

The procedure is performed as an outpatient surgery. The appropriate small joint arthroscopy and MIS equipment should be available. The small joint arthroscopy set up includes either a 1.9-mm or 2.7-mm 30° arthroscope, 2.5-mm shaver, saline irrigation on gravity, and small joint arthroscopic instruments (grasper, biter, and probe). The MIS equipment includes a wedge burr approximately 3.0 mm × 12 to 13 mm (size is system dependent), MIS instruments (beaver blade, periosteal elevator, and soft tissue rasp), and high-speed power system specifically designed for MIS. We prefer to place a nonsterile thigh tourniquet, although this is not routinely inflated. The operative bleeding allows for an additional cooling effect and debris extraction. Additionally, the thigh tourniquet rather than calf allows for appropriate excursion and protection of the extensor hallucis longus (EHL) tendon. General anesthesia or monitored anesthesia care may be used. An ankle block is performed with a 50:50 mix of 0.5% marcaine and 1% lidocaine.

The patient is positioned supine with the heels slightly off the end of the operating table (**Fig. 1**). An ipsilateral hip bump is typically required to position the foot in a more vertical resting position with the toes pointed straight up. The operative heel will rest on and perpendicular to the image intensifier of fluoroscopy machine. We prefer to use the mini C-arm for ease of operation and switching between orthogonal

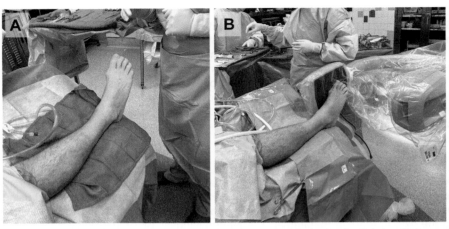

Fig. 1. Patient positioning. (*A*) The patient is positioned with the heels slightly off the end of the operating table. An ipsilateral hip bump is typically required to position the foot in a more vertical resting position with the toes pointed straight up. (*B*) Fluoroscopy is positioned at the end on the table on the patient's right side.

views. For a right-handed surgeon, fluoroscopy is positioned at the end on the table on the patient's right side, regardless of the operative laterality. The opposite is true for a left-handed surgeon, fluoroscopy will always be position at the patient's left side. The limb is prepped and draped in usual sterile fashion and appropriate surgical timeout is performed.

The bony landmarks are palpated, confirmed radiographically, and marked including the metatarsal head, proximal phalanx, joint line, and EHL tendon (**Fig. 2**). The dorsal medial cutaneous nerve (DMCN) should also be marked if identifiable. The medial and lateral arthroscopy portals should be planned at the dorsomedial and dorsolateral aspects of the hallux MTP joint. A separate dorsomedial incision is marked about 2 cm proximal to the dorsomedial arthroscopy portal and MTP joint line. The incision should be medial to the EHL tendon and plantar to the DMCN to avoid iatrogenic injury to either structure. Placing the portal too plantar challenges access to the dorsolateral osteophyte with the burr. When surgeons first start performing this procedure, a slightly larger incision here will protect the skin from excessive hand motions. A 3 to 5-mm dorsomedial stab incision is made using a beaver blade at this location, incising only the skin given proximity of the DMCN. Longitudinal blunt dissection is performed through the soft tissue to the level of the bone with a curved hemostat. A curved periosteal elevator is then used to lift the capsule and dorsal soft tissues off the dorsal osteophyte and create a working space for arthroscopy and the burr (see **Fig. 2**A).

We prefer to first perform an arthroscopic examination and debridement, then cheilectomy with the burr, and finally returning to arthroscopy to ensure adequate resection and removal of all debris. To begin with hallux MTP joint arthroscopy, noninvasive distraction is applied. An arthroscopy distractor is positioned at the foot of the bed (**Fig. 3**A). A 4 × 8 gauze or kerlix is used to create a sleeve around the hallux (in finger trap fashion), which is then attached to the distractor and secured with a hemostat clamp (**Fig. 3**B). A standard dorsomedial portal is created at the joint line. A small incision is made just through the skin medial to the EHL tendon at the level of the joint.

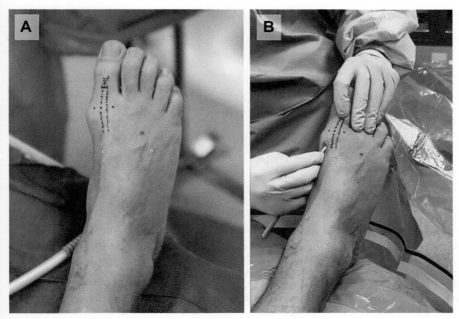

Fig. 2. Landmarks. (*A*) Mark the EHL tendon to avoid iatrogenic injury. Using both clinical palpation and fluoroscopic guidance, mark out the medial and lateral arthroscopy portals at the dorsomedial and dorsolateral aspects of the joint. (*B*) Make a dorsomedial incision about 2 cm proximal to the dorsomedial arthroscopy portal. Through this portal, a curved periosteal elevator is then used to clear the capsule and dorsal soft tissues off the dorsal osteophyte and create a working for the burr space for arthroscopy and the burr.

Blunt dissection is carried deep to the joint capsule and the joint is bluntly entered with the straight hemostat. A blunt trocar and then cannula are placed through the dorsomedial cheilectomy portal, followed by a 2.7-mm arthroscope. Irrigation is to gravity rather than pump. The joint can then be visualized and inspected (**Fig. 4**A). An

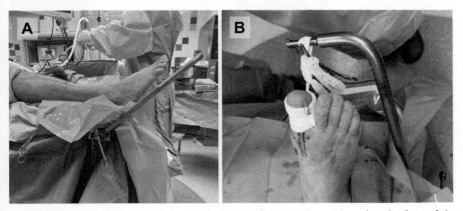

Fig. 3. Arthroscopy distraction. (*A*) An arthroscopy distractor is positioned at the foot of the bed. (*B*) A 4 × 8 gauze or kerlix is used to create a sleeve around the hallux (in finger trap fashion), which is then attached to the distractor and secured with a hemostat clamp.

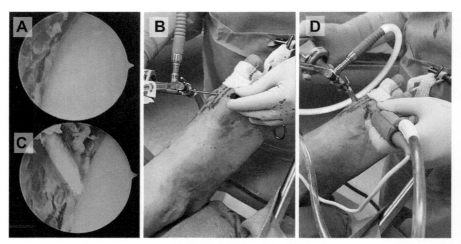

Fig. 4. Portal creation. (*A*) The dorsomedial portal is created in standard fashion. From the medial portal, the dorsolateral aspect of the hallux metatarsal head is visualized as well as hypertrophic synovium. (*B*) A hypodermic needle is placed at the dorsolateral portal site. (*C*) The needle is arthroscopically visualized entering the dorsolateral aspect of the hallux MTP joint capsule. The dorsolateral portal is then created. (*D*) The shaver is then introduced through the dorsolateral working portal.

additional dorsolateral working portal can be made under direct visualization, just lateral to the EHL tendon at the level of the joint. A hypodermic needle is placed at the dorsolateral portal site (**Fig. 4**B). The needle is arthroscopically visualized entering the dorsolateral aspect of the hallux MTP joint capsule (**Fig. 4**C). The dorsolateral portal is then created. This is done in similar technique with a small incision through the skin followed by blunt dissection and penetration into the joint. The shaver is then introduced through the dorsolateral working portal (**Fig. 4**D). The dorsolateral portal is the main working portal used for debridement of the joint. The joint is then inspected with evaluation of the articular surfaces. All hypertrophic synovium is derided (**Fig. 5**).

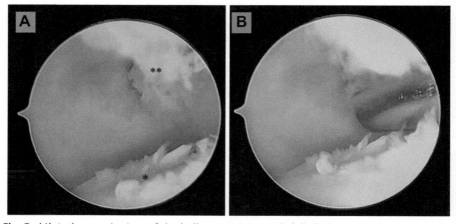

Fig. 5. (*A*) Arthroscopic view of the hallux MTP joint with full-thickness cartilage loss at the dorsal metatarsal head (asterisk) and synovitis (double asterisk). (*B*) The shaver is introduced for debridement of the hypertrophic synovium.

Any chondral changes at the very dorsal aspect of the joint can be disregarded at this point given the planned dorsal cheilectomy. An additional medial midaxial portal can be made for better visualization of the plantar aspect of the metatarsal head if needed. This is made at the distal portion of the MTP joint at the midaxial level using similar technique as prior portals. The arthroscope can also be inserted through this ancillary portal to view the articular surface of the metatarsal head and sesamoids.

Next, the MIS cheilectomy is performed. The wedge burr is introduced through the more proximal dorsomedial incision. The burr is set to high torque and low speed (~6000 rpm) to minimize heat generation. The hallux should be held at either a neutral or a dorsiflexed position to decrease the tension on the EHL and reduce the risk of injuring tendon. The burr is held with an agricultural grip in order to control wedge burr across dorsal metatarsal head (**Fig. 6**). Biplanar fluoroscopy is used to guide the burr and to assess appropriate resection (**Fig. 7**). The burr begins at the base of the osteophyte and is advanced distally (see **Fig. 7**B). Continue across the base until the osteophyte is removed (see **Fig. 7**C). A syringe and angiocatheter is used to apply constant irrigation along the shaft of the burr, soft tissue, and bone to minimize thermal necrosis. Engaging the osteophyte dorsally risks the EHL tendon and is avoided. The amount of resection desired is based on surgeon's preference. Similar to open cheilectomies, the resection involves the osteophyte as well as some degree of the metatarsal head with up to 30% resection of the metatarsal head being acceptable. Greater than 30% of the dorsal metatarsal head removal is not advised because this can destabilize the joint with subluxation of the proximal phalanx.

The burr can also be advanced dorsally over the base of the proximal phalanx to address any dorsal osteophytes at this level. This is performed using a similar technique. Dorsiflexion of the hallux can close down the MTP joint and bring the proximal phalanx to the burr. The arthroscopy portal sites including the dorsomedial, dorsolateral, and medial midaxial may also be used for marginal osteophyte resection. A more proximal dorsolateral portal may also be required for resection of the far lateral osteophytes. However, it is imperative to maintain caution for EHL and DMCN while working through the various portals. The burr will create a bony paste, which requires removal.

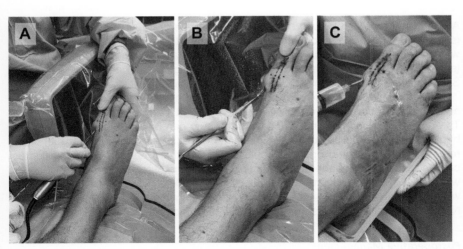

Fig. 6. (*A*) The burr is held with an agricultural grip in order to control the wedge burr across dorsal metatarsal head. (*B*) Removal of resected bone paste with a soft tissue rasp. (*C*) Irrigation of the joint with an angiocatheter and syringe.

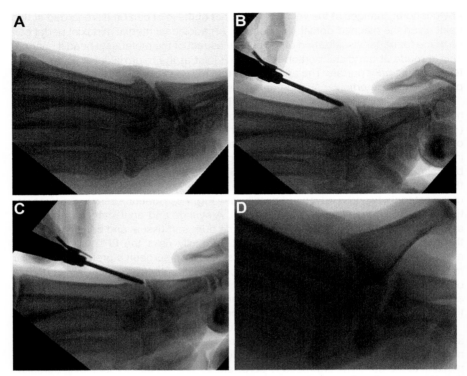

Fig. 7. Lateral fluoroscopic views. (*A*) Precheilectomy image showing dorsal metatarsal head osteophyte. (*B*) Wedge burr initiated at base of spur. (*C*) Completion of osteophyte resection with wedge burr. Note surgeon is maintaining the hallux at a neutral or dorsiflexed position to reduce risk of injuring the EHL. (*D*) Final fluoroscopic evaluation is obtained to verify adequate and even resection, including maximum dorsiflexion view.

A soft tissue rasp can be used to remove soft tissue or capsular bone attachments (see **Fig. 6**B). As the osteophyte is burred, intermittently pause to flush the debris with an angiocatheter and saline while applying manual pressure to express the debris (see **Fig. 6**C). For larger pieces, a small pituitary rongeur can be used for extraction. Saline irrigation should continue until the returned fluid is clear.

At this point, we prefer to reexamine the MTP joint arthroscopically to assess for adequate resection, ensure removal of debris, and perform a final synovectomy. The resection is carefully inspected, and the cuts can be smoothed down with the burr or shaver. Careful fluoroscopic examination must be done to ensure proper debris removal. Any suspected opacity should warrant further debridement. Final fluoroscopy is used to confirm adequate resection and document range of motion of the joint, which should ideally accomplish about 70° of dorsiflexion. Incisions may be closed with wound closure strips or suture. We prefer placing interrupted #3-0 nylon stitches. Nonadherent gauze and a soft, compressive dressing are applied.

Postoperative Management

The patient is placed in a soft dressing and allowed to weight-bear as tolerated in a flat, hard-soled postoperative shoe. Any compressive wrap is removed after 6 hours, and elevation is encouraged for the first 48 to 72 hours. Simple range of motion is encouraged at the hallux MTP joint by grasping the medial and lateral aspects of the proximal phalanx. The bandages are left in place until first follow-up in 10 to 14 days where sutures are removed if the portals are well healed. The patient may then return to normal shoe wear and gentle advancement of activity as their pain and swelling allow. Gradual return to impact and sports is permitted at 4 weeks. Physical therapy is neither routinely recommended nor required.

DISCUSSION
Traditional Open Cheilectomy

Coughlin and Shurnas reported longest follow-up study to date for open cheilectomy with a mean follow-up of 9.6 years.[13] In their 93 patient series, they reported a 92% success rate with open cheilectomy. The study concluded that cheilectomy should be performed for Coughlin and Shurnas Grades I to III hallux rigidus with less than 50% metatarsal head cartilage loss. Similarly, in a series of 197 patients with a mean follow-up of 3.2 years, Bussewitz and colleagues reported an overall success rate of 98.5%.[14] Nicolosi and colleagues reported that 94.83% of their 58 patients stated that they would undergo the same procedure again at a mean of 7.1 years follow-up.[15] More recent studies have also found good long-term results with open cheilectomy, with 69.3% of patients satisfied or very satisfied and 75.1% of patients who would repeat the operation at an average follow-up of 6.6 (5.0–10.9) years.[16] A quantitative literature review analyzed 69 articles discussing operative treatment of hallux rigidus and summarized an average success rate of 74% (range, 40% through 100%) after cheilectomy surgery.[17] There is somewhat contradicting literature on the success of cheilectomy with higher stages of hallux rigidus. However, many authors[15,16,18] pose that cheilectomy is the preferable method as the first-line surgical treatment option for Coughlin and Shurnas Grades I to III hallux rigidus and that outcomes are reliable and favorable irrespective of disease stage.[16]

Minimally Invasive Surgery Cheilectomy

The theoretic benefits of MIS cheilectomy include better cosmesis, reduced wound complications, less soft tissue disruption (which may decrease postoperative scarring and allowing for improved range of motion), and faster recovery. However, further studies are warranted to corroborate these as true benefits over open cheilectomy. In recent literature, MIS cheilectomy demonstrates comparable outcomes to classic open procedures. Although long-term results are lacking compared to classic open cheilectomy, the early to midterm results of MIS cheilectomy from early adopters have been encouraging.

Early results

Pastides and colleagues prospectively followed 47 feet that underwent MIS cheilectomy for grade I to III hallux rigidus with a mean follow-up of 17 months. The authors reported a mean American Orthopaedic Foot and Ankle Society (AOFAS) score of 87.1, improved from 72.1 preoperatively, and 91.4% (32 of 35) patients would undergo the procedure again.[19] Two patients required fusion within this follow-up period, both with Grade III disease. Dawe and colleagues compared open versus MIS cheilectomy reporting satisfaction scores of 9.1 out of 10 and 8.6 out of 10 for MIS and open groups, respectively.[20] Their follow-up was limited to 6 months for the MIS group and 35 months for the open group. They reported one infection in each group and concluded that both procedures had comparable early results. Morgan and colleagues completed an early prospective study comparing open and MIS cheilectomy techniques, again reporting comparable results.[21] The MIS group was followed to a median of 11 months and had an improvement in the Manchester–Oxford Foot Questionnaires (MOXFQ) score from 34 out of 64 preoperatively to 19 out of 64 postoperatively (P < .02). The open group also had a significant improvement in MOXFQ scores. Interestingly, the open group had 3 failures requiring conversion to fusion, whereas the MIS group had none. The authors concluded effectiveness of MIS cheilectomy and similar improvements in pain, function, and social aspects with a potentially lower failure rate.

Midterm results

Teoh and colleagues reported on 98 feet following MIS cheilectomy at a mean of 50 months, demonstrating sustained improvement.[22] Patient-reported outcome improvements including visual analog scale (VAS) score of 8 (from 3 preoperatively) and MOXFQ score of 30.5 (from 58.6 preoperatively). Dorsiflexion was maintained at 69.1° compared to 11.3° preoperatively. The authors also reported a decrease in screening time and fluoroscopy dosage at their center as they performed more MIS cheilectomies, suggesting a learning curve is present.[24,25] Similar outcomes were reported by Hickey and colleagues who followed their group of 36 patients out to a mean of 4.69 years.[23] A total of 83% recommended the procedure again, and 69% had mean postoperative pain improvement. In patients who still reported pain, the mean pain score was 3.4 out of 10. A total of 81% could wear fashionable shoes again. The range of motion was similarly improved. This limited data of midterm follow-up suggest comparable and sustained improvement for MIS cheilectomy.

Arthroscopy

Arthroscopy can be used to accomplish a dorsal cheilectomy with MIS techniques, although early data reported mixed outcomes.[24–26] Debnath and colleagues reported their patients were 95% pain free after arthroscopic hallux rigidus treatment at 2 years.[26] AOFAS scores improved from 43 to 97 and dorsiflexion from 8° to 30°. Two patients required joint sacrificing procedures during the 2-year follow-up period. Glenn and colleagues recently published their results of MIS cheilectomy supplemented with arthroscopy, similar to our described technique.[27] At a mean follow-up of 16.5 months, they demonstrated significantly improved VAS scores, dorsiflexion, and plantar flexion compared to preoperative. They reported no revisions in that period, and only one patient required a fusion at 3 years. Arthroscopic findings included 100% of patients with intra-articular bone debris despite thorough irrigation and 100% had synovitis. They attributed their lack of infection and wound issues as well as sustained outcomes to their more thorough arthroscopic inspection and debridement. Although we agree with the authors regarding the benefits of arthroscopic evaluation, similar outcomes have been reported with and without arthroscopic supplementation.[22,23,27] Recently, this procedure including an MIS cheilectomy and arthroscopy has been described as an in-office in a sterile, wide-awake fashion.[12]

Complications

The most common acute complications of MIS cheilectomy include thermal injury to soft tissue and bone, damage to tendons, nerve injury, wound issues or infections, and iatrogenic cartilage damage.[28] Teoh and colleagues reported 2 wound infections and 2 with delayed wound healing out of 98 patients.[22] Two of these 4 were smokers and all were successfully treated with oral antibiotics and local wound care. This study also reported a 2% incidence of transient nerve palsy and 2 with permanent numbness in the DMCN distribution. No patients had EHL tendon dysfunction. Hickey and colleagues reported 3 out of 36 with numbness in the DCMN and 1 out of 36 with EHL tendon rupture at 6 months postoperatively.[23] Two recent cadaveric studies measured the proximity of the DMCN to the dorsomedial incision.[29,30] The DMCN was found an average of 3.8 mm from the incision and was cut in 2 out of 13 specimens. They identified the DMCN danger zone to be at a third of the length of the metatarsal from the MTP joint. Following these findings, it was suggested that incisions be avoided in the 10 to 2 o'clock positions relative to the medial border of the EHL tendon to avoid the DMCN and the dorsolateral cutaneous nerve.[29,30] Glenn and colleagues reported no DMCN or EHL tendon injuries and no wound issues with their addition of arthroscopy to the procedure.[27] Again, the authors attribute this to a more thorough debridement of bone debris, which can be inflammatory and contribute to wound healing complications or even nerve irritation. Stevens and colleagues performed a retrospective comparison of MIS and open cheilectomy including 38 open and 138 MIS procedures at a mean 3-year follow-up.[31] They reported no infections in the MIS group and no difference in wound complications between the 2 groups (2.6% open vs 3.0% in MIS). The MIS group had one DMCN injury and one EHL tendon rupture, similar to the findings in the other studies. Overall complication rate was higher in the MIS group, although did not reach statistical significance (11.3% vs 2.6% RR 4.29, $P = .076$).

Overall, informal comparison of MIS versus open technique cheilectomy literature demonstrates similar reoperation rates. There are only a couple of studies directly comparing the 2 techniques. In a direct comparison of MIS versus open techniques, Stevens and colleagues reported a higher reoperation rate with MIS cheilectomy compared to open at a mean of 3 years.[31] In their series, only 1 patient in the open group required reoperation while 17 in the MIS group required reoperation (2.6% vs 12.8%, RR 4.86, $P = .059$). Within the MIS group, 10 (7.5%) patients had persistent stiffness and 9 went on to arthrodesis and 1 had an interpositional arthroplasty. All reoperations were attributed to MIS technique errors, mainly the residual bone debris.

Teoh and colleagues reported a similar reoperation rate of 12% in the MIS group (n = 12, 7 arthrodesis, 4 repeat cheilectomy), which they attributed to technique and the learning curve.[22] Interestingly, the groups who performed arthroscopy in conjunction with MIS cheilectomy reported no revision surgeries and only one fusion at 3 years.[23,27] There is some level of learning curve associated with all MIS foot and ankle procedures, and this may contribute to some complications and reoperations. Arthroscopy may be a helpful adjunct to the procedure because it provides a direct view of the articular surface, osteophyte resection, and more thorough washout of bone debris, all of which can minimize complications.[8]

SUMMARY

Hallux MTP joint cheilectomy is a joint-sparing technique that involves resection of the dorsal metatarsal head osteophytes; this may be achieved through minimally invasive and arthroscopic techniques. General indications for MIS cheilectomy are mild-to-moderate hallux rigidus (Grades I–II) with symptomatic dorsal osteophytes causing dorsal impingement and/or shoe wear irritation in those who have failed extensive nonoperative management. The literature confirms equivalent outcomes to open cheilectomy; however, it is somewhat inconsistent regarding superiority. The theoretic benefits of MIS cheilectomy include better cosmesis, reduced wound complications, less soft tissue disruption, and faster recovery.

CLINICS CARE POINTS

Pearls
- A thorough physical examination, particularly assessment of range of motion and dorsal impingement pain, and radiographic evaluation are critical in identifying patients indicated for cheilectomy alone.
- Preoperative counseling is imperative for expectation setting. This should include education on the natural history of hallux rigidus including the risk of progressive arthritis as well as the risks, benefits, and goals of MIS cheilectomy.
- Mark the EHL tendon and DMCN, if able, preoperatively to ensure no iatrogenic injury. Careful incision planning and blunt dissection when creating the portal sites is critical.
- Appropriate position of the proximal dorsomedial portal is critical and should be planned with fluoroscopy to confirm the appropriate trajectory and reach of the burr.
- Lateral osteophytes may require a proximal dorsolateral portal to obtain thorough debridement.
- Fluoroscopy should be used to guide and evaluate thoroughness of resection to the desired depth.
- Close examination of fluoroscopic opacities and thorough arthroscopic debridement are needed to ensure minimal bone debris remains.
- Arthroscopy is used for direct visualization of the cheilectomy resection site, articular surface, synovitis, and to ensure through removal of bone debris.

Pitfalls
- Patients with advanced disease including significant joint space narrowing, positive grind test, resting pain, and pain at midrange of motion are unlikely to receive appropriate relief with cheilectomy alone and joint scarifying procedures may be required.
- Plantar placement of the initial proximal dorsomedial portal will challenge lateral bone resection.
- Thorough irrigation is necessary to avoid thermal injury and necrosis. Avoid high-speed burring and use short bursts with frequent cooling. Avoid large hand movements, which tension the skin. Extend the skin incisions if needed.
- Residual bone debris can incite an inflammatory response leading to wound complications and joint stiffness.
- Plantarflexion of the toe during burring tensions dorsal structures and can increase the risk of iatrogenic damage to the EHL tendon or DMCN.
- Be prepared and comfortable converting to an open procedure at any point. Include this in your preoperative discussion and consent.
- Failure to begin early range of motion and early weight-bearing can lead to increased stiffness.

DISCLOSURE

Dr R. Cerrato: Consultant and Royalties with Stryker, Consultant Vilex, Paid speaker Acumed, Board member MIFAS. Dr A. Fletcher and V. Dr Patel have no disclosures.

REFERENCES

1. Walter R, Perera A. Open, Arthroscopic, and Percutaneous Cheilectomy for Hallux Rigidus. Foot Ankle Clin 2015;20(3):421–31.
2. Coughlin MJ, Shurnas PS. Hallux rigidus: demographics, etiology, and radiographic assessment. Foot Ankle Int 2003;24(10):731–43.

3. Canseco K, Long J, Marks R, et al. Quantitative motion analysis in patients with hallux rigidus before and after cheilectomy. J Orthop Res 2009;27(1):128–34.
4. Hattrup SJ, Johnson KA. Subjective results of hallux rigidus following treatment with cheilectomy. Clin Orthop Relat Res 1988;226:182–91.
5. Coughlin MJ, Shurnas PS. Hallux rigidus. Grading and long-term results of operative treatment. J Bone Joint Surg Am 2003;85(11):2072–88.
6. Keiserman LS, Sammarco VJ, Sammarco GJ. Surgical treatment of the hallux rigidus. Foot Ankle Clin 2005;10(1):75–96.
7. Smith SM, Coleman SC, Bacon SA, et al. Improved ankle push-off power following cheilectomy for hallux rigidus: a prospective gait analysis study. Foot Ankle Int 2012;33(6):457–61.
8. Redfern D, Vernois J, Legré BP. Percutaneous Surgery of the Forefoot. Clin Podiatr Med Surg 2015;32(3):291–332.
9. Schipper ON, Day J, Ray GS, et al. Percutaneous Techniques in Orthopedic Foot and Ankle Surgery. Orthop Clin North Am 2020;51(3):403–22.
10. Razik A, Sott AH. Cheilectomy for Hallux Rigidus. Foot Ankle Clin 2016;21(3):451–7.
11. Hunt KJ. Hallux metatarsophalangeal (MTP) joint arthroscopy for hallux rigidus. Foot Ankle Int 2015;36(1):113–9.
12. Kaplan DJ, Chen JS, Colasanti CA, et al. Needle Arthroscopy Cheilectomy for Hallux Rigidus in the Office Setting. Arthrosc Tech 2022;11(3):e385–90.
13. Coughlin MJ, Shurnas PS. Hallux rigidus. J Bone Joint Surg Am 2004;(Pt 2):119–30, 86-A Suppl 1.
14. Bussewitz BW, Dyment MM, Hyer CF. Intermediate-term results following first metatarsal cheilectomy. Foot Ankle Spec 2013;6(3):191–5.
15. Nicolosi N, Hehemann C, Connors J, et al. Long-Term Follow-Up of the Cheilectomy for Degenerative Joint Disease of the First Metatarsophalangeal Joint. J Foot Ankle Surg 2015;54(6):1010–20.
16. Sidon E, Rogero R, Bell T, et al. Long-term Follow-up of Cheilectomy for Treatment of Hallux Rigidus. Foot Ankle Int 2019;40(10):1114–21.
17. Maffulli N, Papalia R, Palumbo A, et al. Quantitative review of operative management of hallux rigidus. Br Med Bull 2011;98:75–98.
18. Cetinkaya E, Yalcinkaya M, Sokucu S, et al. Cheilectomy as a First-Line Surgical Treatment Option Yields Good Functional Results in Grade III Hallux Rigidus. J Am Podiatr Med Assoc 2016;106(1):22–6.
19. Pastides P, El Sallakh S, Charalambides C. Minimally Invasive Cheilectomy for the Treatment of Grade I to III Hallux Rigidus: A Prospective Study Reporting on Early Patient Outcome. Tech Foot Ankle Surg 2014;13:98–102.
20. Dawe EJC, Ball T, Annamalai S, et al. Early results of minimally invasive cheilectomy for painful hallux rigidus. J Bone Joint Surg B 2012;94-B:18.
21. Morgan S, Jones C, Palmer S. Minimally invasive cheilectomy (MIS): functional outcome and comparison with open cheilectomy. J Bone Joint Surg Br 2012;94(93).
22. Teoh KH, Tan WT, Atiyah Z, et al. Clinical Outcomes Following Minimally Invasive Dorsal Cheilectomy for Hallux Rigidus. Foot Ankle Int 2019;40(2):195–201.
23. Hickey BA, Siew D, Nambiar M, et al. Intermediate-term results of isolated minimally invasive arthroscopic cheilectomy in the treatment of hallux rigidus. Eur J Orthop Surg Traumatol 2020;30(7):1277–83.
24. van Dijk CN, Veenstra KM, Nuesch BC. Arthroscopic surgery of the metatarsophalangeal first joint. Arthroscopy 1998;14(8):851–5.

25. Iqbal MJ, Chana GS. Arthroscopic cheilectomy for hallux rigidus. Arthroscopy 1998;14(3):307–10.
26. Debnath UK, Hemmady MV, Hariharan K. Indications for and technique of first metatarsophalangeal joint arthroscopy. Foot Ankle Int 2006;27(12):1049–54.
27. Glenn RL, Gonzalez TA, Peterson AB, et al. Minimally Invasive Dorsal Cheilectomy and Hallux Metatarsal Phalangeal Joint Arthroscopy for the Treatment of Hallux Rigidus. Foot Ankle Orthop 2021;6(1). 2473011421993103.
28. Walther M, Chomej P, Kriegelstein S, et al. [Minimally invasive cheilectomy]. Oper Orthop Traumatol 2018;30(3):161–70.
29. Teoh KH, Haanaes EK, Alshalawi S, et al. Minimally Invasive Dorsal Cheilectomy of the First Metatarsal: A Cadaveric Study. Foot Ankle Int 2018;39(12):1497–501.
30. Malagelada F, Dalmau-Pastor M, Fargues B, et al. Increasing the safety of minimally invasive hallux surgery-An anatomical study introducing the clock method. Foot Ankle Surg 2018;24(1):40–4.
31. Stevens R, Bursnall M, Chadwick C, et al. Comparison of Complication and Reoperation Rates for Minimally Invasive Versus Open Cheilectomy of the First Metatarsophalangeal Joint. Foot Ankle Int 2020;41(1):31–6.

Cartiva
A Review of the Best Evidence

Timothy Daniels, MD, FRCSC[a,b], Caroline Cristofaro, MBChB[a,b],
Mansur Halai, MBChB, MRCS, FRCS (Tr & Orth)[a,b,*]

KEYWORDS

- Cartiva • Hemiarthropasty • Polyvinyl • Hydrogel

KEY POINTS

- Level I evidence exists showing that the Cartiva is a safe and efficacious treatment of hallux rigidus while conserving some range of motion postoperatively.
- Cartiva can be used in the spectrum of treatments for hallux rigidus, not jeopardizing a future arthrodesis of the first metatarsophalangeal joint.
- There are technique pearls that one should consider when using the Cartiva. These include keeping it extra proud or adding a Moberg-Akin osteotomy.

SUMMARY OF OUTCOMES

Baumhauer and colleagues published the only level I evidence comparing first metatarsophalangeal (MTP) arthrodesis with Cartiva for the treatment of hallux rigidus, and therefore deserves a more detailed analysis.[1] This multicenter, noninferiority 2:1 randomized controlled trial (RCT) was conducted within the United States, Canada, and the United Kingdom. Patients aged 18 years or older with symptomatic (preoperative visual analog score [VAS] > 40) hallux rigidus grade 2 or greater, using the Coughlin and Shurnas Classification, were included. The primary outcome was "successful" if the following criteria were met: improvement from baseline in VAS pain of 30% or greater at 12 months, maintenance of function from baseline in Foot and Ankle Ability Measure (FAAM) sports subscore at 12 months; and absence of major safety events. They enrolled 47 patients into the arthrodesis (control) group and 147 into the Cartiva (intervention) group. Noninferiority of the Cartiva implant, compared with arthrodesis, was defined as less than the equivalence limit (−15%). Significant improvements in VAS and FAAM were demonstrated following Cartiva at 12 and 24 months. Rates of revision procedures were similar between the intervention and control groups (11.2% and 12.0%, respectively) with 9.2% of patients undergoing conversion to

a Department of Orthopaedics, University of Toronto, Canada; b Department of Orthopaedics, St Michael's Hospital, Toronto, Canada
* Corresponding author. Suite 800, 55 Queen Street East, Toronto, Ontario M5C 1R6, Canada.
E-mail address: Mansur.Halai@Unityhealth.to

Foot Ankle Clin N Am 29 (2024) 485–493
https://doi.org/10.1016/j.fcl.2023.11.004
1083-7515/24/Published by Elsevier Inc.

foot.theclinics.com

arthrodesis (equivalent to published revision rates of nonunion following first MTP arthrodesis). Goldberg subsequently evaluated the RCT data and found no statistically significant differences in success rates for either group when data were stratified by any of the following: grade of hallux rigidus, degree of preoperative hallux valgus, extent of preoperative ROM, patient demographics, duration of symptoms, earlier MTPJ surgery status, and preoperative VAS pain score.[2]

Using the same cohort from the Baumhauer and colleagues RCT, Glazebrook demonstrated statistically significant reduced surgical and anesthesia times in patients undergoing this polyvinyl alcohol (PVA) hemiarthroplasty.[3] They found that the mean operative time for hemiarthroplasty was 35 ± 12 minutes and 58 ± 21 minutes for arthrodesis ($P < .001$). They also reported that the mean anesthesia time was 28 minutes shorter with hemiarthroplasty ($P < .001$). A subsequent article followed a subset of 112 patients from the Baumhauer and colleagues RCT cohort for 2 to 5 years postoperatively and found that 7.6% of patients underwent implant removal and conversion to arthrodesis. Daniels demonstrated an implant survivorship of 96% with their subset of 27 patients from the Baumhauer and colleagues RCT and had been treated at a Canadian site and present for in-person follow-up.[4] One patient underwent conversion to arthrodesis for persistent pain.

Brandao published a case series from the United Kingdom of 55 patients who underwent Cartiva for moderate-to-severe hallux rigidus and were followed up for a mean of 21 months.[5] Postoperative FAAM activities of daily living scores showed statistical improvement. One patient underwent conversion to arthrodesis. Similarly, a further article compared an athletic subset of this cohort (30 patients who underwent Cartiva and participated in sporting activities) with 23 patients who underwent cheilectomy (5 with mild, 10 with moderate, and 8 with severe hallux rigidus). They found no statistically significant difference between postoperative FAAM sport scores, and return to function/sport times were also comparable.[6,7]

Hoskins and colleagues also compared 31 cheilectomy patients to 21 who underwent Cartiva.[8] They found that patients with Cartiva had statistically significant greater improvement in both American Orthopedic Foot and Ankle Society (AOFAS) scores and dorsal ROM when compared with those who underwent cheilectomy. Two patients with Cartiva and 6 patients who underwent cheilectomy complained of mild pain at final follow-up. Similarly low rates of revision were reported in a retrospective cohort study of 103 patients who had undergone Cartiva (52 who also underwent an Moberg osteotomy) by Eble. Once again, patients who underwent Cartiva had significant improvements across all patient-reported outcome measures information systems (PROMIS) domains at 26 months postoperatively. These scores were lower in patients who had already undergone a previous procedure such as a previous Cartiva, cheilectomy, or Moberg osteotomy. Eble also found that patients who underwent concurrent Moberg osteotomy had less pain postoperatively.[9] Only 2 (1.9%) patients underwent revision surgery, one conversion to arthrodesis and the other a revision Cartiva. Both had higher pain interference and pain intensity scores postoperatively compared with patients who did not undergo a revision procedure.

Zanzinger published an implant survival rate of 93% in their cohort of 44 patients who underwent first MTP joint arthroplasty with Cartiva at 12 months.[10] Both VAS and AOFAS scores improved significantly postoperatively ($P < .05$). Notably, ROM at the first MTP joint did not show significant improvement (preoperative: 31°, postoperative: 32°). Lee also reported favorable results in a cohort of 96 patients who underwent Cartiva. VAS pain scores demonstrated significant improvement from preoperative baseline ($P < .001$).[11] However, 12.5% of patients reported no improvement with Cartiva. Two patients (2.1%) required revision to arthrodesis, and 2 patients underwent tibial sesamoidectomy for refractory sesamoid pain. The latter is, of course, a potential problem with both arthrodesis and arthroplasty.

Higher complication rates have also been reported. Shimozono published a small case series of 11 patients, 3 of who underwent revision surgery in the form of implant fixation with fibrin glue.[12] They also noted a 90% subsidence rate on postoperative radiographs at a mean follow-up of 20.9 months. Despite the relatively high rate of revision, their cohort had a statistically significant VAS improvement ($P=.01$). An and colleagues studied radiographic as well as clinical outcomes of 16 patients with 18 Cartiva implants who had ongoing symptoms postoperatively at a mean of 13 months.[13] They demonstrated significant progressive loss of the joint space ($P < .001$).[13] All cases had edema surrounding the implant and many had subsided below the subchondral bone of the MT head.[13] Engasser and colleagues published a retrospective cohort study in 2020. They reported that 72.5% of patients responded that they would "definitely" or "probably" have the surgery again, whereas 27.5% would not.[14] There were 10 patients who underwent revision surgery (16.9%) with the majority (n = 7) converted to arthrodesis. They demonstrated statistically significant improvement in preoperative to postoperative VAS and FAAM scores.[14]

Chrea and colleagues published a retrospective case control study with 72 patients who had undergone Cartiva in addition to a Cheilectomy and Moberg (CM) osteotomy compared with those who underwent only CM osteotomies.[15] Both groups demonstrated a statistically significant improvement in PROMIS scores postoperatively but patients with only CM osteotomies had statistically higher physical function and lower pain intensity scores when compared with patients with Cartiva.[15] The Cartiva group had 3 revisions and 3 infections, whereas the CM osteotomy group had one conversion to arthrodesis and no infections. They concluded that, although results with Cartiva plus CM osteotomies had good outcomes, equivalent or better outcomes could be achieved with CM osteotomies only.[15]

Cassinelli and colleagues published a case series of 60 patients undergoing Cartiva with a single surgeon at their institution.[16] Notably, their rate of previous procedures was high (23%). Average PROMIS scores were improved at 15 months clinical follow-up; however, a significant proportion of patients fell into the "mild dysfunction" range for physical function and "mild pain interference," with 27% of patients reporting that they were "very unsatisfied" and 11% who would have preferred a fusion.[16] One in 5 patients required a revision procedure: lysis of adhesions (4), Moberg osteotomy (1), and implant exchange with bone grafting for impinging soft tissue or implant subsidence (3), and conversion to fusion (5).[16] Thirty-eight percent of patients reported being unsatisfied with their outcome postoperatively. They concluded that although outcomes improved from baseline scores with Cartiva, patients should be well informed of surgical risks and complications.[16]

CAUSES OF FAILURE

Akoh and colleagues analyzed all adverse events reported to the Federal Drug Agency (FDA) from 2010 to 2018 and found 15 total event reports for Cartiva. They reported 5 incidences of implant subsidence, 2 of component fracture, 2 infections, 5 inflammation, and 1 dislocation but excluded incomplete reports.[17] The FDA's Manufacturer and User Facility Device Experience use inflammation as a common patient problem code and, given that these are voluntary public reports, there is no standardized clinical symptomology for each problem code. Metikala and colleagues published a similar study on FDA-reported adverse events of Cartiva but from 2016 to 2019.[18] They found 16 reports of implant subsidence, 9 of broken or fragmented devices, 4 cases of infection, 3 with surrounding eroded bone or fractured MT, 1 foreign body re-action, and 16 reports were "unspecified."[18] Eleven of the 16 subsided implants un-derwent revision, and 5 reports did not include information regarding outcome. Of the total 49 adverse reports, 10 underwent conversion to arthrodesis, 4 had a revision Cartiva, and the remaining 35 had either debridement and reimplantation of the same Cartiva (2) or removal of the Cartiva with an alternative revision procedure.

Shi and colleagues conducted a retrospective radiographic review of 27 consecu-tive patients who underwent first MTP joint hemiarthroplasty with Cartiva and measured their preoperative and postoperative joint space area. Similar to previous reported findings, they found that the joint space area significantly decreased in the first 5 to 12 weeks following surgery.[12,16–19] There have been no studies to the authors' knowledge demonstrating causation between implant subsidence and poor patient outcome; however, increased subsidence leads to implant loosening and can cause decreased bone stock, which makes revision surgery challenging. **Fig. 1** shows a technique to revise a Cartiva due to subsidence, maintaining motion.

The most reported salvage technique is conversion to arthrodesis, and its indication is typically pain not resolved by nonoperative means. There are limited evidence pub-lished specifically describing salvage procedures for Cartiva implants. Davies and col-leagues have published a detailed surgical technique on conversion from Cartiva to arthrodesis while illustrating 3 clinical cases successfully completed at their center.[20] First, infection must be ruled out by appropriate preoperative workup (ie, serologic in-flammatory markers) followed by imaging to assess bone stock. The Cartiva implant requires little bone resection given its small size (8–10 mm) and therefore autologous bone graft or allograft is often not required.[20] Davies and colleagues describe using cancellous bone autograft from the calcaneus in defects less than 15 mm but also advocate for the gold standard of iliac crest bone graft in larger defects.[20] In cases of revision, the previous incision is used, and the medial and lateral capsule is released to allow dislocation of the first MTP joint and removal of the implant. A bone lever can be used to extricate the Cartiva from the MT head. Tissue samples should be sent for culture to evaluate for infection. Joint surfaces are prepared as per surgeon prefer-ence (Davies and colleagues advocate for cannulated small joint reamers) and the remaining bone void is measured. After placing bone graft if needed, the joint is

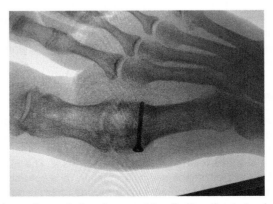

Fig. 1. Intraoperative radiograph showing a revision Cartiva, due to implant subsidence. The implant was removed, the reaming void backfilled with calcaneal auto graft, and then a raft horizontal 2.7-mm screw placed to prevent further subsidence.

stabilized with either 2 crossed screws or a dorsal plate and the capsule is repaired.[20] One of the 3 cases illustrated had a larger, conical bone void secondary to a subsided implant that had been present in the patient for more than 5 years. This was treated with calcaneus autograft in addition to reamings. The authors report that the revision is not technically challenging, and most cases involve minimal or modest bone loss.[20]

PATIENT SELECTION, TECHNIQUE PEARLS, AND ADJUNCT PROCEDURES

Cartiva is indicated for patients with symptomatic (VAS $\geq$40), moderate-to-advanced hallux rigidus who have failed nonoperative management (ie, stiff soled shoe/carbon footplate, cortisone injection, nonsteroidal anti-inflammatories) and have good bone stock ($\geq$2 mm bone present to surround implant).[1,21] Younger and colleagues emphasize that patients must be symptomatic at the first MTP joint and not at the sesamoidal region because sesamoid arthritis symptoms will not be alleviated with Cartiva. Substantial hallux valgus deformity, multiple comorbidities, osteoporotic bone, and significant first MT anatomic deformity are contraindications to hemiarthroplasty.[21,22] Preoperative ROM must be 10° or greater to 15° of dorsiflexion beyond neutral, preferably 30° to 40°.[21]

Younger and colleagues and Glazebrook and colleagues have described the surgical approach for Cartiva in detail.[21–23] A standard dorsal incision just medial to the extensor hallucis longus (EHL) tendon is used, the EHL is retracted laterally, the dorsal medial cutaneous nerve is protected, and the capsule is incised longitudinally. The MTP joint is then dislocated with flexion of the great toe, and the Cartiva sizing device is placed perpendicular to the MT shaft. The sizing device is then used to determine whether the 8-mm or 10-mm prosthesis should be used. A rim of bone 1 to 2 mm thick must be intact surrounding the implant to ensure stability. A guidewire is placed through the sizer 15 to 10 mm down the first MT shaft, the sizer is then removed, and fluoroscopy is used to confirm the guidewire's central placement orthogonally. Care must be taken to ensure the guidewire is central because eccentric reaming can lead to eccentric placement of the implant and resultant shearing/MT fracture.[21] A reamer is subsequently advanced over the guidewire with irrigation to prevent bone necrosis. Ensure not to ream excessively because the implant should be at least 2 mm proud in the MT shaft.[1] The implant is then loaded into the delivery tube (convex side up) with sterile saline to lubricate. The implant is introduced into the reamed space of the MT shaft via the delivery tube in a single smooth motion. The implant is then confirmed to protrude 1.5 to 2 mm (Baumhauer and colleagues even advocate for 1.5–2.5 mm given evidence of early subsidence) and the joint is brought through ROM.[1,21] After copious irrigation, the capsule is closed followed by skin.

There are tips and tricks published to assist surgeons in the more technically demanding aspects of the procedure. First, surgeons should consider underreaming (leaving implant 1.5–3.0 mm proud) to prevent the implant from being placed too deeply in the case of slightly eccentric reaming.[21,24] This is illustrated through a dorsal approach in **Fig. 2**. Glazebrook and colleagues advise removal of the Cartiva and packing with reamings should the implant be less than 1 mm proud from the MT shaft.[22] They also advocate for the removal of osteophytes only after the Cartiva is in situ to preserve bone.[21,22] Younger and colleagues describe performing a sesamoid release and shortening or plantarflexion osteotomies of the first MT in cases where it is pathologically long or excessively dorsiflexed, respectively, to manage MTP joint stiffness.[21] If dorsiflexion ROM remains suboptimal, or slight plantarflexion of the proximal phalanx remains after the Cartiva is inserted, Younger and colleagues advocate for consideration of a concomitant Moberg osteotomy.[21] This osteotomy is shown in **Fig. 3**A with the corresponding radiograph in **Fig. 3**B.

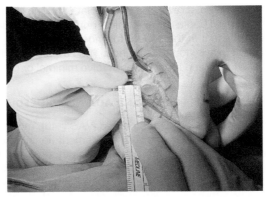

Fig. 2. First MTP joint showing the Cartiva implant, via a dorsal approach, lying 3 to 4 mm proud.

Postoperative care is typically weight-bearing as tolerated in a postoperative shoe with compressive footwrap to keep the first MTP joint in 5° to 10° of dorsiflexion and no restrictions in ROM once the surgical incision is healed (around 2–3 weeks).[21] Pain relief begins at 3 months and improves up to 6 to 9 months postoperatively. Perhaps, this long period of potential improvement should be explained to the patient, to manage expectations on their recovery.[21]

SHOULD IT BE USED INSTEAD OF FUSION?

There has been level I evidence published supporting the claim that first MTP hemiarthroplasty with Cartiva is a safe and efficacious treatment of hallux rigidus while conserving some ROM postoperatively.[1] Multiple retrospective cohort studies and case series also support these findings.[5,8–10] Equally, there have been level IV studies with poorer patient outcomes following Cartiva with high rates of concerning radiographic findings, including implant subsidence, osteolysis, and MT erosion.[16,19,25] Guyton and colleagues also published a reanalysis of the data in the Baumhauer and colleagues RCT and found that by altering basic assumptions within the data, the results of Cartiva fall below the noninferiority margin.[26] The lower bound of the

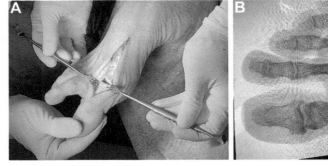

Fig. 3. Moberg-Akin osteotomy of the proximal phalanx, in conjunction with a Cartiva. (*A*) The clinical picture after the osteotomy and screw placement, with (*B*) showing the corresponding radiograph.

95% confidence interval fell below the noninferiority margin of −15.0% when applying any of the following criteria to the data[1]: including cases of asymptomatic radiographic failures in the "failure" category[2] including isolated implant removal as a "failure"[3] using a Visual Analog Scale (VAS) pain threshold of less than 30 as a "success" as opposed to a 30% reduction in VAS pain score.[26]

The PVA hemiarthroplasty is still a relatively novel implant, and our knowledge of complications is limited to the early term and midterm. Evidence has demonstrated significant levels of implant subsidence radiographically; however, there have been no studies directly linking these radiographic findings to patient outcomes. Additionally, Glazebrook and colleagues has demonstrated that patients undergoing Cartiva removal and conversion to arthrodesis for failure exhibited outcome measure scores statistically such as those of the primary arthrodesis cohort at 2 years. This would suggest that failed treatment with Cartiva does not "burn a bridge" to having good outcome with a revision arthrodesis.[27]

It is difficult to definitively state whether a Cartiva implant should be used instead of arthrodesis. Considering contradictory evidence, the authors advocate for open, honest discussion with patients and clear communication regarding published outcomes. Patient selection is crucial, and perhaps, this only comes with surgical experience in doing both procedures. Although patients with a Cartiva may be able to continue activities such as yoga or wearing heeled shoes with the preserved ROM, they must be counseled that pain relief may take longer and the risk of revision may be higher than with a fusion. In addition, more research is needed in the coming years regarding long-term outcomes of Cartiva.

CLINICS CARE POINTS

- Patient selection is paramount. Ensure there is at least 10° of preoperative range of motion (ROM) at the MTP joint and less than 10° of Hallux valgus before considering the Cartiva.
- Immediate ROM and weight-bearing is to be encouraged.
- Consider adjuncts to implantation such as leaving the implant proud 3 mm, backfilling the reamed void with autograft or performing a Moberg-Akin osteotomy.
- According to the RCT, the patient will continue to improve up to 1 year postoperatively. Do not consider a revision fusion before this time point.

DISCLOSURE

The authors certify that neither (s)he nor any members of his or her immediate family have any commercial associations (such as consultancies, stock ownership, equity interest, patent/licensing arrangements, and so forth) that might pose a conflict of interest in connection with the submitted article.

REFERENCES

1. Baumhauer JF, Singh D, Glazebrook M, et al. Prospective, randomized, multi-centered clinical trial assessing safety and efficacy of a synthetic cartilage implant versus first metatarsophalangeal arthrodesis in advanced hallux rigidus. Foot Ankle Int 2016 -05;37(5):457–69.
2. Goldberg A, Singh D, Glazebrook M, et al. Association between patient factors and outcome of synthetic cartilage implant hemiarthroplasty vs first metatarsophalangeal

joint arthrodesis in advanced hallux rigidus. Foot Ankle Int 2017 -11;38(11): 1199–206.

3. Glazebrook M, Younger ASE, Daniels TR, et al. Treatment of first metatarsophalangeal joint arthritis using hemiarthroplasty with a synthetic cartilage implant or arthrodesis: a comparison of operative and recovery time. Foot Ankle Surg 2018 -10;24(5):440–7.

4. Daniels TR, Younger ASE, Penner MJ, et al. Midterm outcomes of polyvinyl alcohol hydrogel hemiarthroplasty of the first metatarsophalangeal joint in advanced hallux rigidus. Foot Ankle Int 2017;38(3):243–7.

5. Brandao B, Aljawadi A, Hall A, et al. Cartiva case series: the efficacy of the cartiva synthetic cartilage implant interpositional arthroplasty at one year. J Orthop 2020; 20:338–41.

6. Brandao B, Aljawadi A, Poh ZE, et al. Comparative study assessing sporting ability after Arthrodesis and Cartiva hemiarthroplasty for treatment of hallux rigidus. J Orthop 2020;18:50–2.

7. Brandao B, Hall A, Aljawadi A, et al. Joint sparing management of hallux rigidus: Cartiva SCI vs cheilectomy a comparative review. J Orthop 2020;21:401–5.

8. Hoskins T, Barr S, Begley B, et al. Synthetic cartilage implant hemiarthroplasty versus cheilectomy for the treatment of hallux rigidus. Eur J Orthop Surg Traumatol 2023;33(6):2567–72.

9. Eble SK, Hansen OB, Chrea B, et al. Clinical outcomes of the polyvinyl alcohol (PVA) Hydrogel implant for hallux rigidus. Foot Ankle Int 2020;41(9):1056–64.

10. Zanzinger C, Harrasser N, Gottschalk O, et al. One-year follow-up results with hydrogel implant in therapy of hallux rigidus: case series with 44 patients. Z für Orthop Unfallchirurgie 2022;160(4):414–21.

11. Lee W, Wang C, Prat D, et al. Patient satisfaction following hallux rigidus treatment with a synthetic cartilage implant. Foot Ankle Spec 2021 -03;-26. 19386400211001993.

12. Shimozono Y, Hurley ET, Kennedy JG. Early failures of polyvinyl alcohol hydrogel implant for the treatment of hallux rigidus. Foot Ankle Int 2021 -03;42(3):340–6.

13. An TW, Cassinelli S, Charlton TP, et al. Radiographic and magnetic resonance imaging of the symptomatic synthetic cartilage implant. Foot Ankle Int 2020;41(1): 25–30.

14. Engasser WM, Coetzee JC, Ebeling PB, et al. Patient-reported outcomes and early complications after synthetic cartilage device implantation. Foot Ankle Orthop 2020;5(3). 2473011420930691.

15. Chrea B, Eble SK, Day J, et al. Comparison Between Polyvinyl Alcohol Implant and Cheilectomy With Moberg Osteotomy for Hallux Rigidus. Foot Ankle Int 2020;41(9):1031–40.

16. Cassinelli SJ, Chen S, Charlton TP, et al. Early Outcomes and Complications of Synthetic Cartilage Implant for Treatment of Hallux Rigidus in the United States. Foot Ankle Int 2019;40(10):1140–8.

17. Akoh CC, Chen J, Kadakia R, et al. Adverse events involving hallux metatarsophalangeal joint implants: Analysis of the United States Food and Drug Administration data from 2010 to 2018. J Foot Ankle Surg 2021;27(4):381–8.

18. Metikala S, Mahmoud K, O'Connor K,M, et al. Adverse events related to cartiva hemiarthroplasty of first metatarsal: an analysis of reports to the united states food and drug administration. Foot Ankle Spec 2022;15(2):113–8.

19. Rosas K, Hurley ET, Kennedy JG. Early failures of polyvinyl alcohol hydrogel implant for the treatment of hallux rigidus. Foot Ankle Orthop 2020 November 6;5(4). 2473011420S00414.

20. Davies MB, Roberts VI, Chadwick C, et al. Revision of synthetic cartilage implant hemiarthroplasty of the great toe to metatarsophalangeal joint arthrodesis: technique and indications. Tech Foot Ankle Surg 2020 March;19(1):48.

21. Younger ASE, Glazebrook MA, Daniels TR, et al. First metatarsophalangeal joint polyvinyl alcohol hydrogel implant hemiarthroplasty: current operative technique. Tech Foot Ankle Surg 2022 March;21(1):30.

22. Glazebrook MA. Cartiva hemi arthroplasty for treatment of hallux rigidus: surgical technique, evidence and tips and tricks. Fuß & Sprunggelenk 2019;17(1):28–32.

23. Younger ASE, Baumhauer JF. Polyvinyl alcohol hydrogel hemiarthroplasty of the great toe: technique and indications. Tech Foot Ankle Surg 2013;12(3):164.

24. Baumhauer JF, Daniels T, Glazebrook M. New technology in the treatment of hallux rigidus with a synthetic cartilage implant hemiarthroplasty. Orthop Clin North Am 2019;50(1):109–18.

25. Shi E, Todd N, Rush S, et al. First metatarsophalangeal joint space area decreases within 1 month after implantation of a polyvinyl alcohol hydrogel implant: a retrospective radiographic case series. J Foot Ankle Surg 2019 -11;58(6): 1288–92.

26. Guyton GP. Philosophies of surgical care are embedded in outcome studies: an illustrative reanalysis of the cartiva motion trial. Foot Ankle Int 2022;43(10): 1364–9.

27. Glazebrook M, Baumhauer J, Davies M. Revision of implant to great toe fusion: did we "burn a bridge" with a synthetic implant hemiarthroplasty? Foot & Ankle Orthopaedics 2017;2. 2473011417S0000.

Metatarsophalangeal Arthroplasty in Hallux Rigidus

Rohan Bhimani, MD, MBA, Sameh A. Labib, MD*

KEYWORDS

- Hallux valgus • Hallux rigidus • First metatarsophalangeal joint • Arthrodesis
- Cheilectomy • Interpositional arthroplasty

KEY POINTS

- The article describes hallux rigidus (HR)–relevant clinical presentations and classifications that guide management.
- The article discusses HR nonoperative versus operative management with results.
- The article details pros and cons of hallux metatarsophalangeal arthroplasty, current techniques, and long-term results.

 Video content accompanies this article at http://www.foot.theclinics.com.

INTRODUCTION

Hallux rigidus (HR) is the most common degenerative condition of the foot that limits range of motion of the first metatarsophalangeal joint (MTPJ) and leads to pain with motion.[1–4]

ANATOMY

The anatomy of the first MTPJ plays an important role in the development of HR.[5] The dorsoplantar diameter of the first metatarsal head is smaller than its transverse diameter.[6] In addition, the articular surface of the metatarsal head is functionally divided into superior and inferior fields, with superior field having a larger convex dome than its phalangeal counterpart.[7] The inferior field, on the other hand, is larger than the superior and is divided into 2 sloped sesamoids articulations by a ridge.[7] The ridge is

Funding: The author(s) received no financial support for the research, authorship, and/or publication of this article.

Foot and Ankle Division, Department of Orthopaedic Surgery, Emory University School of Medicine, Emory Orthopedics, 1968 Hawks Lane, # 200, Atlanta, GA 30329, USA

* Corresponding author.

E-mail address: slabib@emory.edu

located at the intersection of the medial two-third and lateral one-third of the articular surface, allowing for more room for a larger tibial sesamoid.

The proximal phalanx at the first MTPJ has a large transversely oriented concave articular surface that matches the first metatarsal head. The articular surface of the proximal phalanx has multiple tubercles for insertions of tendons from the flexor and extensor hallucis brevis, adductor and abductor halluces, and intrinsic foot muscles.[7] Along the plantar aspect of the first metatarsal, there are 2 sesamoids that are located within the plantar plate capsuloligamentous complex and articulate with the corresponding articulations of the metatarsal head. The tibial sesamoid is larger and more ovoid in shape, whereas the fibular sesamoid is smaller, rounder, and more proximally located.[8] Additionally, the plantar plate is an important component of the first MTPJ capsuloligamentous complex, providing attachment for ligaments and tendons both medially and laterally. It plays an important role in the stability of the first MTPJ. The plantar plate is attached to the first metatarsal 1.73 cm proximal to the MTPJ line and to the proximal phalanx, 0.3 mm distal to the joint line.[8]

SURGICAL MANAGEMENT

Numerous surgical treatment options are available when nonoperative measures fail. These techniques fall into 2 categories: joint sparing techniques and joint sacrificing techniques. The procedure chosen will depend on the degree of degenerative changes in the joint, the patient's motivation, goals, and ultimate expectations for the surgery. The purpose of surgery is to relieve pain, enhance function, keep the first MTPJ stable, and improve overall quality of life.

Surgical treatment options are cheilectomy, interpositional arthroplasty, osteotomies, first MTPJ arthrodesis, and hemiarthroplasty and total joint arthroplasty. Our article will focus on arthroplasty of the first MTPJ.

Partial or total joint arthroplasty is a surgery designed to relief pain while preserving some mobility of the first MTPJ. Historically, great toe arthroplasty was performed with silicone implants. These implants were primarily designed as soft tissue spacers but were unable to withstand the high loads placed on them by the first MTPJ. That usually leads to a high failure rate due to reactive bone response and silicone implant fracture.[9] Double-stemmed silicone implants with grommets were later introduced to improve fixation and reduce silicone wear. However, silicone debris, foreign body reactions with osteolysis, implant failure issues, and systemic silicone complications such as silicone lymphadenitis, brain cancer, and alopecia were reported with the use of these implants.[9,10] This led to the development of metal implants as an alternative for hallux MTPJ resurfacing. Hallux MTPJ hemiarthroplasty or total joint arthroplasty is contraindicated in patients with active or previous history of infection, inadequate bone stock, neuropathic foot, advanced sesamoid arthritis, inflammatory arthritis, metal allergy, and accompanying severe hallux valgus.

Hemiarthroplasty

Hemiarthroplasty involves the insertion of a metallic implant into either the metatarsal head or the proximal phalanx (**Fig. 1**). This procedure has the advantage of causing less surgical morbidity in the form of decreased first MTPJ pain and improved motion. Until the introduction of metatarsal hemiarthroplasty in 2005 (HemiCAP, Arthrosurface, Franklin, MA), hemiarthroplasty for HR was limited to the phalangeal surface. Theoretically, a phalangeal hemiarthroplasty implant was thought to act as a spacer, ensure maintenance of toe length, and was placed on the phalanx that carries less weightbearing of the first MTPJ, and thus lower risk of failure. However, the caveat

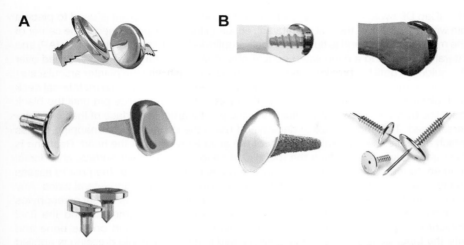

Fig. 1. First metatarsophalangeal joint hemiarthroplasty implants. (*A*) Hemiarthroplasty metallic implants inserted on the proximal phalanx. (*B*) Hemiarthroplasty metallic implants inserted on the metatarsal head.

to using the phalangeal implant was not addressing the first metatarsal head where degeneration was predominant and often resulted in continued joint stiffness, pain, and subsequent implant loosening.[11,12] This led to the development of first metatarsal hemiarthroplasty devices.

The HemiCap, the metatarsal hemiarthroplasty implant, was introduced in 2005 as a 2-part implant (HemiCAP, Arthrosurface, Franklin, MA, USA). The articular surface is a cap-like metatarsal head made of cobalt-chromium (CoCr) with a Morse taper fixation into a titanium (Ti)-tapered cannulated screw. The HemiCap DF (Arthrosurface, Franklin, MA, USA) is a second-generation implant with a dorsal flange designed with double radii of curvature built into the dorsal slope of the cap at 12° of dorsiflexion of the first MTPJ to improve phalangeal roll-off with dorsiflexion of the first metatarsal head.[13,14] Metatarsal hemiarthroplasty or the HemiCap procedure requires minimal bone resection for implantation of this device and is indicated in patients with first MTPJ arthritis, predominantly involving the metatarsal head, to relieve pain while preserving range of motion.[15]

Surgical procedure

A longitudinal dorsal approach medial to the extensor hallucis longus (EHL) tendon is utilized to access the first MTPJ. The subcutaneous tissue is carefully dissected to avoid injury to the dorsomedial cutaneous branch of the superficial peroneal nerve and the dorsal joint capsule is exposed. The EHL tendon is retracted laterally, and the capsule is entered longitudinally ensuring that full thickness capsular flaps are raised off the bone both medially and laterally. To ensure complete visualization of the joint, including the sesamoids, the collateral ligaments, the sesamoid suspension ligaments, and capsule are completely released. The crista of the metatarsal sesamoid articulation serves as a landmark for sizing of the implant and its visualization is critical. However, any damage to the articulation surface of sesamoid should be avoided. In advanced HR, the insertions of the plantar plate, collaterals and flexor hallucis brevis tendon, are often released from the proximal phalanx to achieve intraoperative 90° of dorsiflexion of the first MTPJ.

After exposing the joint, the metatarsal head is resurfaced using techniques described by the manufacturer. The description that follows is derived from the

HemiCap DF system technique guide. A drill guide from the implant is used to place a pin within the shaft of the first metatarsal, ensuring that pin is positioned in the center of the metatarsal shaft and is fluoroscopically confirmed on both anteroposterior (AP) and lateral views. Using a cannulated double-step drill, the metatarsal head is drilled over the guide pin until the proximal shoulder of the drill is flush with the plantar articular surface of the metatarsal head. A corkscrew tap is then utilized to tap the metatarsal neck until black laser line. The taper post is then passed over the guide pin until the black laser line over the screwdriver is flush with the plantar articular surface of the first metatarsal head. The implant size is determined using the contact probe mapping guides which measure the articular geometry of the articular surface of the head. Reaming is then undertaken to resurface the metatarsal head using articular surface and dorsal reamers to match the implant. The trial implant is then attached to the post to assess range of motion and adequacy of coverage on dorsal, medial, and lateral sides. Any excess bone on medial and lateral sides of the implant, as well as dorsal osteophytes over the proximal phalanx, is removed. The trial implant is removed, and the final implant is impacted until the articular component is firmly seated on the bone and into the taper post. The wound is finally closed in layers. A sterile dressing is applied which is left intact until follow-up. Patients are permitted to heel weight bear in a postoperative shoe and their sutures are removed in about 2 weeks from surgery.

Outcomes

Mixed results have been reported on hemiarthroplasty of the first metatarsal head. Currently, there are no recent studies on the HemiCap DF, and all research has been done with the first-generation implant. In a prior retrospective study, Voskuijl and Onstenk[16] evaluated outcomes in 58 primary arthrodesis and 36 hemiarthroplasties with an average 4-year follow-up. They reported no difference in the American Orthopedic Foot and Ankle Society Hallux Metatarsophalangeal Interphalangeal (AOFAS-HMI) score between the 2 groups (77.5 ± 18.5 and 77.8 ± 12.0 in the arthrodesis and arthroplasty groups, respectively). Moreover, they found that the number of reoperations did not differ between these 2 groups, but patients treated with hemiarthroplasty had higher satisfaction rates. Similarly, Beekhuizen and colleagues[17] retrospectively assessed outcomes in 47 primary arthrodesis and 31 hemiarthroplasties with an average 8.3-year follow-up. The authors found AOFAS-HMI score to be higher in the hemiarthroplasty group (72.8 ± 14.5 vs 89.7 ± 6.6 in the arthrodesis and hemiarthroplasty groups, respectively). In addition, the patients had an earlier return to sporting activities, a higher satisfaction rate after hemiarthroplasty, and would recommend this procedure more often. Furthermore, they reported the number of re-surgeries and the overall crude costs were similar for both procedures.

By contrast, Raikin and colleagues retrospectively compared clinical and radiographic outcomes of 21 feet with hemiarthroplasties using the BioPro implant (phalangeal side implant) and 27 feet that underwent first MTPJ arthrodesis for HR.[18] In the hemiarthroplasty group, they found plantar cutout of the prosthetic stem in 8 feet, dorsal subsidence in 13 implants, and an overall 24% percent revision rate at an average 79.4-month follow-up. In the arthrodesis group, on the other hand, they had no revisions at an average 30-month follow-up. Moreover, in the hemiarthroplasty group, decreased AOFAS-HMI scores and satisfaction level and higher Visual Analogue Scale (VAS) pain scores were seen compared with arthrodesis patients. The authors found that the mean AOFAS-HMI score significantly increased postoperatively from 36.1 to 83.8 (93.1%) of 90 points in the arthrodesis group and from 35.6 to 71.8 (71.8%) in the hemiarthroplasty group. Additionally, they reported rates of implant failure, defined as the need for fusion or revision hemiarthroplasty, of 4.8%, 14.3%, and

23.8% at 9, 12, and 18 months postoperatively based on the Kaplan-Meier survivorship analysis. Similarly, Gheorghiu and colleagues[19] found decreased patient satisfaction and range of motion and 58% subsidence in 11 patients (12 feet) who underwent hemiarthroplasty at an average 47 months follow-up.

Total Joint Arthroplasty

The historic success of metal on polyethylene implants in the hip and knee has led to the hope of similar success in the first MTPJ. Unfortunately, earlier generation implants did not regain motion and have failed at a high rate mainly due to loosening.[20] Subluxation and loosening were also observed in the subsequent generation of implants that used press-fit ceramic or metal components (Ti/CoCr) to secure the implant in the bone.[21] Currently, the fourth-generation implants in use have the bearing surface now secured by press-fit or threaded stems with a Morse taper. In patients with advanced stage of HR with significant degenerative changes on both metatarsal head and phalangeal surface, total joint arthroplasty can be a good surgical option especially in those who wish to be pain-free and preserve first MTPJ motion (**Fig. 2**). In the United States, several total toe arthroplasty implants are available:
Three-component systems.

1. ToeMotion (Arthrosurface, Franklin, MA, USA)
2. Movement Great Toe (Integra, Plainsboro, New Jersey, USA)
3. ReFlexion (OsteoMed, Irving, TX, USA)

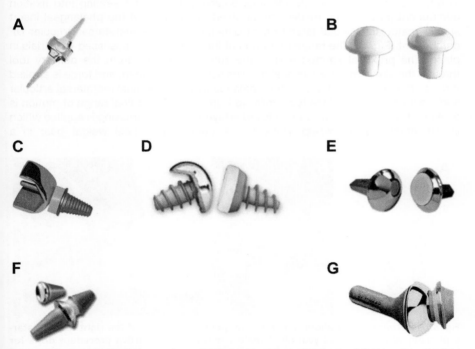

Fig. 2. First metatarsophalangeal total joint arthroplasty implants. (*A*) Swanson flexible hinge total toe implant. (*B*) MOJE 'press-fit' ceramic implant. (*C*) ToeMobile implant. (*D*) ToeMotion implant. (*E*) Bio-Action great toe implant. (*F*) Toefit-plus implant. (*G*) ReFlexion total toe implant.

Two-component systems.

1. ToeMobile (Merete, New Windsor, NY, USA)

Surgical procedure

The first MTPJ is approached via a longitudinal dorsal approach medial to the EHL tendon as described in the hemiarthroplasty section. Releasing the collateral ligaments, sesamoid suspension ligaments on the metatarsal side, and plantar plate, collaterals, and flexor hallucis brevis tendon on the proximal phalanx side, allows complete visualization of the joint as well as 90° of dorsiflexion at the first MTPJ (**Fig. 3**, Video 1). The manufacturer's recommended methods are used to resurface the joint after the joint has been exposed. The description that follows is for the Toe-Motion system. "The metatarsal head is prepared, and trial is implanted as described for the HemiCap DF. The medial exostosis of the hallux and the spurs all around the prosthesis are removed. Using the pin drill guide, a 1.5 mm guide pin is placed in the center along the axis of the proximal phalanx and confirmed radiographically on AP and lateral views (**Fig. 4**). Reamer is passed over the guide pin and reaming is performed until the depth indicator is flush to the phalangeal articular surfaces on the medial, lateral, and plantar sides (see **Fig. 4**). A corkscrew tap is then utilized to tap the area until depth indicator is flush to the level of the original (before reaming) phalangeal articular surface. The guide pin is then removed, and the phalangeal fixation component is advanced in the tapped pilot hole using a Hex driver until the component is fully seated in phalangeal socket and confirmed fluoroscopically. Trial inserts are used to determine the final phalangeal insert for seating into fixation component (**Fig. 5**). The medial lateral offset dimensions of the phalangeal insert should match the medial lateral offset dimensions of the metatarsal articular DF component (**Fig. 6**). The range of motion of the first MTPJ is assessed with trials in place. The proximal knotted end of the suture is passed from the delivery tool through the slot in the Hex Driver shaft. The suture is tensioned, and force is applied through the delivery tool to seat the phalangeal insert. The final metatarsal articular surface implant is then inserted similar to HemiCap DF and final range of motion is evaluated (Video 2). The wound is closed in layers. A sterile dressing is applied which is left intact until follow-up. Patients are permitted to heel weight bear in a

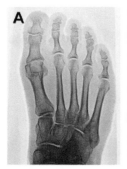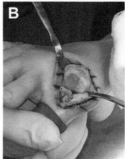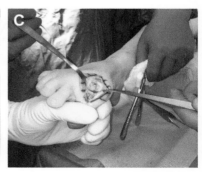

Fig. 3. Anteroposterior radiograph and intraoperative findings of the right first metatarsophalangeal joint in a 54-year-old female 7 months after Cartiva procedure done for hallux rigidus. (*A*) Anteroposterior radiograph of the right foot demonstrating first metatarsophalangeal joint arthritis with interpositional implant. (*B*) and (*C*) Intraoperative photo showing a painful Cartiva implant that was removed prior to replacement with toe MTP implant.

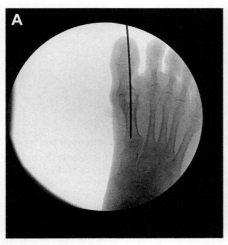
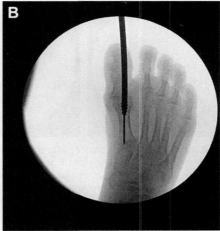

Fig. 4. Intraoperative fluoroscopic images during metatarsal preparation during total toe implantation in the right first metatarsophalangeal joint. (*A*) Intraoperative anteroposterior (AP) fluoroscopic image demonstrating insertion of guide pin within the shaft of the first metatarsal. (*B*) Intraoperative anteroposterior (AP) fluoroscopic image demonstrating drilling of the metatarsal head over the guide pin.

postoperative shoe and their sutures are removed in about 2 weeks from surgery (**Fig. 7**, Video 3).

Outcomes

Total joint arthroplasty for the first MTPJ has also yielded mixed outcomes. Erkocak and colleagues[22] evaluated the results of the three-component ToeFit-Plus prosthesis (Plus Orthopedics AG, Switzerland) in 26 feet at an average 29.9 months follow-up. In their retrospective study, they found significant improvement in the AOFAS score, VAS pain scores, and first MTPJ range of motion. Surprisingly, there was no radiological

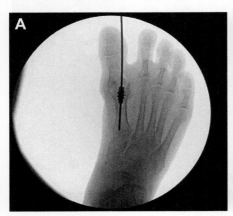
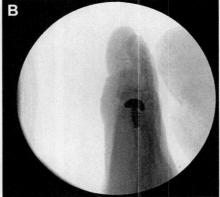

Fig. 5. Intraoperative fluoroscopic images during metatarsal implant insertion during total toe implantation in the right first metatarsophalangeal joint. (*A*) Intraoperative anteroposterior (AP) fluoroscopic image demonstrating insertion of the taper post over the guide pin within the shaft of the first metatarsal. (*B*) Intraoperative anteroposterior (AP) fluoroscopic image demonstrating trial implant attached to the taper post.

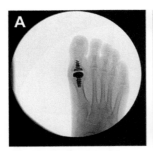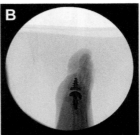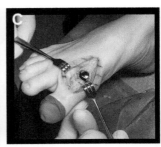

Fig. 6. Intraoperative fluoroscopic and clinical images after insertion of implants during total toe implantation in the right first metatarsophalangeal joint. (*A*) Intraoperative anteroposterior (AP) fluoroscopic image demonstrating insertion of the total toe implants. (*B*) Intraoperative lateral fluoroscopic image demonstrating insertion of the total toe implants. (*C*) Total Toe prosthesis implanted through a dorsal approach.

loosening or need for revision required for any of the patients during the follow-up period. Bartak and colleagues[23] assessed outcomes of total joint arthroplasty using ToeFit-Plus prosthesis in 19 feet at an average 24 month follow-up. They reported improvement in Kitaoka score and range of motion at the first MTPJ. However, 3 cases had radiographic evidence of asymptomatic osteolysis around both the phalangeal and the metatarsal component.

In contrast, a retrospective study by Gupta and colleagues[24] evaluated long-term results of the ToeFit-Plus replacement in 55 cases at an average 11.2-year follow-up. The authors reported 21% revision rate with 23% of the cases reporting continued pain and stiffness. A systematic review by Brewster and colleagues[25] compared functional outcomes of arthrodesis and total joint replacement of the first MTPJ. They found no difference in the median postoperative AOFAS-HMI score between the 2 groups (83/100 for total joint arthroplasty and 82/100 for arthrodesis). In addition,

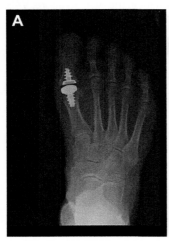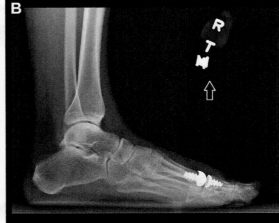

Fig. 7. Radiographic images of right foot in a 54-year-old female 10 weeks after total toe implantation. (*A*) Anteroposterior (AP) radiograph of right foot demonstrating first metatarsophalangeal total joint implant in good position with no breakage or subsidence. (*B*) Lateral radiograph of right foot demonstrating first metatarsophalangeal total joint implant in good position with no breakage or subsidence.

they reported a 7% median revision rate in joint replacement group and 0% for arthrodesis group. Similarly, Titchener and colleagues[26] compared clinical and radiological outcomes with ToeFit-Plus replacement in 86 toes at an average 33 months follow-up. They found a revision of rate of 24% in their patient group. Additionally, radiographic lucency was seen in 25 joints and 7 joints were frankly loose. These radiographic changes were mainly seen on the phalangeal side.

COMPLICATIONS OF FIRST METATARSOPHALANGEAL JOINT ARTHROPLASTY

Despite the newer designs, multiple complications have been reported with continued MTPJ pain and stiffness including implant failure, aseptic loosening, infection, lucency, instability, transfer metatarsalgia, and sesamoid impingement.[18,19,25,26]

Finally, a recent study by Akoh and colleagues[27] examined the US Food and Drug Administration's Manufacturer and User Facility Device Experience database to review voluntary reported adverse event reports for approved implants within the United States. Among 64 MTPJ device adverse events reported, the most common reason for reported adverse events was component loosening (34.4%), infection (14.1%), component fracture (9.4%), inflammation (9.4%), allergic reactions (9.4%), periprosthetic fracture (7.8%), component malposition (6.3%), dislocation (3.1%), size mismatch (3.1%), dislocation (3.1%), nerve problems (1.6%), and impingement (1.6%).

SUMMARY

The first MTPJ arthroplasty is a viable surgical treatment for HR. Individuals who desire pain relief from HR but are unwilling to accept the loss of motion that arthrodesis entails now have options due to newer implants and techniques. Despite good outcomes of implants in the literature, reports of increased complication rates, uncertain results, and poor survivorship rates have led orthopedic surgeons to be wary of using implant arthroplasty. Additionally, the potential for sizable bone loss due to the procedure in the first place made management of failed arthroplasty an extremely challenging salvage procedure. Further work with larger cohorts and longer follow-up studies are needed to establish a more definitive conclusion about arthroplasty in HR.

CLINICS CARE POINTS

- HRis a common and disabling arthritic condition that affects active individuals.
- Correct diagnosis and classifications are essential for proper management.
- Hallux MTP arthroplasty is a viable option that can improve pain and maintain function. It also has procedure-specific long-term limitations that need to be discussed with prospective patients.

DISCLOSURE

The author(s) declared no potential conflicts of interest with respect to the research, authorship, and/or publication of this article.

SUPPLEMENTARY DATA

Supplementary data related to this article can be found online at https://doi.org/10.1016/j.fcl.2023.12.003.

REFERENCES

1. Shurnas P, Coughlin M. Arthritic conditions of the foot. *Surgery of the Foot and Ankle.* Philadelphia: Mosby Elsevier; 2007. p. 805–921.
2. Coughlin MJ, Shurnas PS. Hallux rigidus. Grading and long-term results of operative treatment. J Bone Joint Surg Am 2003;85(11):2072–88.
3. Shurnas PS. Hallux rigidus: etiology, biomechanics, and nonoperative treatment. Foot Ankle Clin 2009;14(1):1–8.
4. Hamid KS, Parekh SG. Clinical Presentation and Management of Hallux Rigidus. Foot Ankle Clin 2015;20(3):391–9.
5. Coughlin MJ, Shurnas PS. Hallux rigidus: demographics, etiology, and radiographic assessment. Foot Ankle Int 2003;24(10):731–43.
6. Sarrafian SK. Anatomy of the foot and ankle: descriptive, topographic, functional. Lippincott Williams & Wilkins; 1993.
7. Lucas DE, Hunt KJ. Hallux Rigidus: Relevant Anatomy and Pathophysiology. Foot Ankle Clin 2015;20(3):381–9. https://doi.org/10.1016/j.fcl.2015.04.001.
8. Lucas DE, Philbin T, Hatic S. The plantar plate of the first metatarsophalangeal joint: an anatomical study. Foot Ankle Spec 2014;7(2):108–12.
9. Granberry WM, Noble PC, Bishop JO, et al. Use of a hinged silicone prosthesis for replacement arthroplasty of the first metatarsophalangeal joint. J Bone Joint Surg Am 1991;73(10):1453–9.
10. Husson G, Herrinton LJ, Brox WT, et al. A cohort study of systemic and local complications of toe prostheses. Am J Orthop (Belle Mead NJ) 2003;32(12):585–92.
11. Giza E, Sullivan M, Ocel D, et al. First metatarsophalangeal hemiarthroplasty for hallux rigidus. Int Orthop 2010;34(8):1193–8.
12. Townley CO, Taranow WS. A metallic hemiarthroplasty resurfacing prosthesis for the hallux metatarsophalangeal joint. Foot Ankle Int 1994;15(11):575–80.
13. Butterworth ML, Ugrinich M. First Metatarsophalangeal Joint Implant Options. Clin Podiatr Med Surg 2019;36(4):577–96.
14. San Giovanni T. Arthrosurface HemiCAP Resurfacing. In: Weisel S, editor. Operative techniques in orthopaedic surgery. Lippincott Williams & Wilkins; 2016.
15. Carpenter B, Smith J, Motley T, et al. Surgical treatment of hallux rigidus using a metatarsal head resurfacing implant: mid-term follow-up. J Foot Ankle Surg 2010; 49(4):321–5.
16. Voskuijl T, Onstenk R. Operative Treatment for Osteoarthritis of the First Metatarsophalangeal Joint: Arthrodesis Versus Hemiarthroplasty. J Foot Ankle Surg 2015;54(6):1085–8.
17. Beekhuizen SR, Voskuijl T, Onstenk R. Long-Term Results of Hemiarthroplasty Compared With Arthrodesis for Osteoarthritis of the First Metatarsophalangeal Joint. J Foot Ankle Surg 2018;57(3):445–50.
18. Raikin SM, Ahmad J, Pour AE, et al. Comparison of arthrodesis and metallic hemiarthroplasty of the hallux metatarsophalangeal joint. J Bone Joint Surg Am. Sep 2007;89(9):1979–85.
19. Gheorghiu D, Coles C, Ballester J. Hemiarthroplasty for Hallux Rigidus: Mid-Term Results. J Foot Ankle Surg 2015;54(4):591–3.
20. Weil LS, Pollak RA, Goller WL. Total first joint replacement in hallux valgus and hallux rigidus. Long-term results in 484 cases. Clin Podiatry 1984;1(1):103–29.
21. Cook E, Cook J, Rosenblum B, et al. Meta-analysis of first metatarsophalangeal joint implant arthroplasty. J Foot Ankle Surg 2009;48(2):180–90.

22. Erkocak OF, Senaran H, Altan E, et al. Short-term functional outcomes of first metatarsophalangeal total joint replacement for hallux rigidus. Foot Ankle Int. Nov 2013;34(11):1569–79.
23. Barták V, Popelka S, Hromádka R, et al. [ToeFit-Plus system for replacement of the first metatarsophalangeal joint]. Acta Chir Orthop Traumatol Cech 2010; 77(3):222–7.
24. Gupta S, Masud S. Long term results of the Toefit-Plus replacement for first metatarsophalangeal joint arthritis. Foot (Edinb) 2017;31:67–71.
25. Brewster M. Does total joint replacement or arthrodesis of the first metatarsophalangeal joint yield better functional results? A systematic review of the literature. J Foot Ankle Surg 2010;49(6):546–52.
26. Titchener AG, Duncan NS, Rajan RA. Outcome following first metatarsophalangeal joint replacement using TOEFIT-PLUS™: A mid term alert. Foot Ankle Surg 2015;21(2):119–24.
27. Akoh CC, Chen J, Kadakia R, et al. Adverse events involving hallux metatarsophalangeal joint implants: Analysis of the United States Food and Drug Administration data from 2010 to 2018. Foot Ankle Surg 2021;27(4):381–8.

Arthrodesis for Hallux Rigidus

Antoine S. Acker, MD[a,b],*, Jeffrey Liles, MD[a], Mark E. Easley, MD[a]

KEYWORDS

- Hallux rigidus • First • MTP fusion • Arthrodesis

KEY POINTS

- First metatarsophalangeal (MTP) joint arthrodesis has been a cornerstone in treating hallux rigidus since the 1950s and remains an excellent option.
- Arthrodesis is recommended for patients with advanced joint degeneration.
- Several constructs have been reported in the literature with high union rates. It is our preference to use either dual plating or combination dorsal plate with lag screw.
- Optimal positioning is crucial for success, and malunion is likely underreported in the literature.

 Video content accompanies this article at http://www.foot.theclinics.com

INTRODUCTION

Hallux rigidus is a degenerative arthritic condition affecting the first metatarsophalangeal (MTP) joint. This condition results in reduced joint mobility, pain, and the development of osteophytes. It ranks as the second most common ailment targeting the first MTP joint after hallux valgus and stands as the predominant form of arthritis in the foot.[1,2] Women are more prone to this condition than men, and it often manifests bilaterally.[1,2] Many patients, before seeking professional medical intervention, attempt to alleviate symptoms using nonsteroidal anti-inflammatory drugs, but as the disease advances, these methods generally prove ineffective.[3] Initial treatments usually lean toward conservative approaches, resorting to surgical methods when conservative measures fail.[3] There is a wide array of surgical options available, ranging from joint arthrodesis to joint-sparing techniques such as osteotomies or replacements.[4,5] Each option has utility based on the desired outcomes and patient-specific characteristics.

[a] Department of Orthopaedic Surgery, Duke University Medical Center, Durham, NC 27710, USA; [b] Centre of Foot and Ankle Surgery, Clinique La Colline, Geneva, Switzerland
* Corresponding author. Department of Orthopaedic Surgery, Duke University, 5601 Arringdon Park Dr, Morrisville, NC 27560-5643.
E-mail address: antoine.acker@duke.edu

Foot Ankle Clin N Am 29 (2024) 507–520
https://doi.org/10.1016/j.fcl.2024.02.008
1083-7515/24/© 2024 Elsevier Inc. All rights reserved.

First MTP joint arthrodesis is a surgical procedure in which the head of the first metatarsal and the base of the proximal phalanx are surgically placed in contact with each other to promote bony bridging and eliminate motion through the first MTP joint. Originally described in 1894 as a procedure for severe hallux valgus, Clutton recommended using an ivory peg to help eliminate motion.[6] Various constructs have since been described, but one of the earliest detailed techniques was published by McKeever. The series was composed of 56 feet in which a stainless steel screw with a washer was inserted from the proximal phalanx, across the MTP joint, and seated in the metatarsal shaft.[7]

During the following decades, the first MTP arthrodesis was regarded as the gold standard to treat end-stage hallux rigidus.[8–10] Multiple techniques have since been developed to improve fusion rates and outcomes ranging from Kirschner wires, lag screws, lag screws with dorsal plating, compression staples, or various combinations of different techniques.[11]

This article highlights our preferred methods of first MTP arthrodesis as well as tips and special considerations based on underlying foot pathology.

PATIENT SELECTION

The ideal candidate for the first MTP joint arthrodesis is one with low functional demand and a grade 4 or a grade 3 arthritic joint with less than 50% remaining cartilage.[12] A patient with high functional demand and more than 50% of cartilage and no pain at mid-range motion does well with conservative management or joint-sparing procedures that are out of the scope of this discussion. It is hard to characterize patients and determine which treatment algorithm they fall into; as such, there is no consensus on the optimal treatment of these patients. Shariff and Myerson emphasize the importance of assessing the motion of the first MTP joint under simulated weight-bearing conditions to identify "functional hallux rigidus." They recommend arthrodesis or treating patients with this condition with arthroplasty.[4]

APPROACH

Three approaches are described in the literature for first MTP arthrodesis: dorsal, medial, and arthroscopic.[13] With the dorsal approach, the extensor hallucis longus tendon is retracted laterally to expose to articular capsule. The medial approach offers direct visualization of the joint, ensuring precise alignment, but care should be made to identify and protect the dorsomedial cutaneous nerve to prevent irritation. A longitudinal capsular incision is made, and the capsule is reflected dorsally. Some investigators expressed concern about the blood supply to the capsule and metatarsal head citing this as a downfall to this approach.[14]

Hodel and colleagues reviewed arthroscopic and percutaneous technique and reported satisfactory results but could not drew a clear superiority of this technique over open approaches.[13] There is heterogeneity in the functional outcome measures reported after arthroscopic arthrodesis; however, some studies have reported improved outcome scores compared to open first MTP arthrodesis.[15]

PREPARATION

Widely accepted today, Rose first suggested to prepare the first MTP joint surfaces with conical reamers in 1950 in an unpublished series reported by Wilson.[16] This was done with a convex and concave reamer on the distal metatarsal head and the proximal phalanx, respectively (**Fig. 2**). Wilson reported that significant soft tissue preparation is necessary to use the reamers and "*the direction of the cylindrical reaming determines, for the most part, the final position of the arthrodesis.*"[16] We believe that conical reamers allow for high degrees of adjustability in a 3 dimensional plane. It is our experience that care should be taken in patients with poor bone quality to avoid unnecessary removal of excess bone and fragmentation of the bone. This can be done by removing large osteophytes that may catch the reamer prior to reaming, keeping the reamer on full speed, and progressing slowly and circumferentially at the preparation sites.

Planar cuts require less extensive dissection; however, it is our experience that the correction and final positioning of the first MTP is more challenging with this technique. With this technique, a first cut is made on the proximal phalanx perpendicular to its anatomic axis (**Fig. 1**), and then a second cut is made on the metatarsal head based on the desired final position. In case of severe deformity or short first metatarsal, this procedure is technically more challenging and can result in shorting of the first ray which can lead to overloading of the lesser metatarsals.[17,18]

It is our preference to perform joint preparation with the cup and cone reamer technique (**Fig. 2**). We believe that flat cut preparation is technically demanding and any malposition requires additional cuts. With the cup and cone reamer technique, there is a large amount of bony contact given the large surface area. Additionally, pronation/supination as well as varus/valgus positioning is easily adjusted to put the toe in optimal position without requiring additional bony resection (see **Fig. 2**).

The arthroscopic and minimally invasive approach requires the use of a burr to prepare the articular surfaces and is not our preferred choice of technique.[13]

There is no superiority of one open approach over the other; however, the dorsal approach allows easier exposure for the use of cups and reams. The medial approach allows better visualization of the orientation of cuts in relation to dorsiflexion. The minimally invasive approach involves the exclusive use of screws.

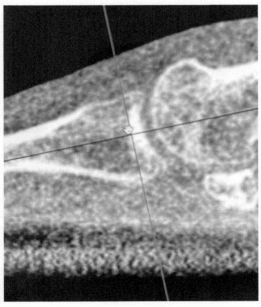

Fig. 1. Demonstration of proximal phalanx cut perpendicular to the anatomic axis (*blue line*).

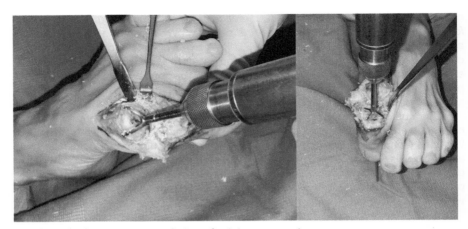

Fig. 2. Cup and cone reamer technique for joint preparation.

Positioning of the First Metatarsophalangeal Arthrodesis

Regarding positioning of the first MTP for arthrodesis, little has changed since the first publication describing this technique. McKeever wrote: "*to determine the angle of arthrodesis between the first metatarsal and the proximal phalanx (...), this is determined by pressing the first metatarsal as close as possible to the second metatarsal and then putting the first and the second toe side by side (...) the angle varies according to the anticipated function. In men it will be approximately 15 to 20 degrees of extension. In women who habitually wear shoes with medium heel it will be from 15 to 25 degrees.*"[7]

One exception since the original publication is the advocation of increased extension of the first MTP in the sagittal plane for women compared to men.

Metatarsus primus elevatus is a common finding among patients with hallux rigidus.[10,19,20] Coughlin and Shurnas reported a normalization of the first metatarsal declination angle.[12] Previously reported optimal dorsiflexion allows the tip of the great toe to touch a flat plate used to simulate weight-bearing and elevation above the simulated weight-bearing plate of a finger width (5 mm).[17]

Lewis and colleagues reported that a proximal shift of an arthrodesis plate was correlated with an increase of dorsiflexion.[21] The effect was greater with a 10° precontoured arthrodesis plate than with a straight plate. Leaseburg and colleagues found a correlation between the bend in the plate and the first MTP angle, but the toe-to-floor distance did not rely exclusively on plate angle. Therefore, the surgeon must consider the anatomy of each patient to optimize the sagittal position of the arthrodesis.

Correct positioning of the toe prior to implanting hardware is critical for successful outcomes in first MTP arthrodesis. We have found that excessive retraction of the medial skin can lead to pronation deformity of the toe. To help prevent deformity during retraction, we advocate for increased provisional fixation prior to hardware implantation (**Fig. 3**).

In terms of rotation, we believe that the toe should be in a neutral position. This allows for uniform contact of the toe tuft on a weight-bearing surface. This is best assessed by viewing the rotation of the toe looking down the axis of the toe from the tip (**Fig. 4**). The toe should also be in a neutral position rather than a slight valgus position.

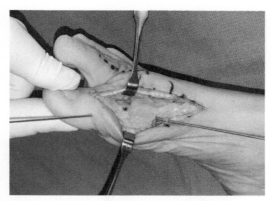

Fig. 3. Increasing provisional fixation can prevent deformity during retraction and hardware implantation.

In the sagittal plane, it is our preferred technique to use a simulated weight-bearing plate for assessment of toe position. We believe that the sesamoids should contact the plate and the tuft should just contact the plate in a way that a freer can pass easily between the plate and the tuft of the distal phalanx (**Fig. 5**). Underlying foot deformity can affect the sagittal positioning of the toe. In a patient with a cavus deformity, proper positioning of the toe may seem elevated when not in a stimulated weight-bearing position. However, under stimulated weight-bearing conditions, the tuft of the toe should just touch the plate as previously described.

An example of this technique can be seen from Supplemental Video 1.

Unlike with hallux valgus, the surgeon has no influence on the rotation of the metatarsal, but the ideal positioning of the hallux is not discussed in the literature. A common clinical finding among patient with hallux rigidus is hyperkeratosis on the medial aspect of the hallux at the level of the interphalangeal (IP) joint suggesting mechanical overload.

Fixation method

Many techniques of fixation are available including the use of oblique lag alone, lag screw combined with dorsal plate fixation, dorsal plate fixation alone, crossed Kirschner wires, or combinations of various techniques.[10,19]

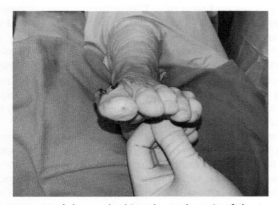

Fig. 4. Rotation assessment of the toe looking down the axis of the toe with ideal neutral rotation.

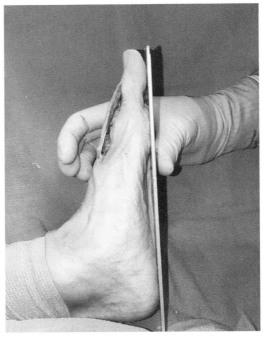

Fig. 5. Simulated weight-bearing technique in which the tip of the great toe just touches the plate.

Dorsal plating with lag screws offers the most biomechanically stable construct but also is associated with the highest cost.[19] An example of this can be seen from **Fig. 6**.

A review from Haimes and colleagues showed that dorsal plating has a mean cost of $603.57 compared to $374.05 for screw fixation alone. A survey from 2013 to 2018 reported an average additional cost of $1500 with the use of locking plates compared to nonlocking plates without any additional changes in the overall nonunion rate (10.1%).[22]

A retrospective study by Claassen and colleagues examined the effect of locking versus nonlocking plates on fusion rate. They retrospectively reviewed data from 60 patients who underwent first MTP arthrodesis with a lag screw and either a titanium dorsal locking plate or a titanium dorsal nonlocking plate. They reported higher nonunion rate with titanium locked plates (17.2%) compared to nonlocking stainless steel plates (11.7%).[23] Interestingly, this nonunion rate is higher than other studies which reported nonunion rates ranging from 2% to 10%.[24,25] The investigators suggest that placing the lag screw after the locking screw could explain this higher nonunion rate. A recent systematic review confirmed the superiority of dorsal plating with lag screw compared to other techniques.[26]

A cadaveric biomechanical study by Schafer and colleagues examined the use of compression staples in first MTP arthrodesis with unsatisfactory results with 15 out of 16 specimens failing cyclic loading in this study.[27]

Despite its lower fusion rate, satisfactory clinical outcomes are reported with screw fixation. Nevertheless, it is not predictable which patient will need a revision due to a painful nonunion and which patient will not. Therefore, we strongly advocate to choose the construct with the highest fusion rate when performing the first MTP arthrodesis. In

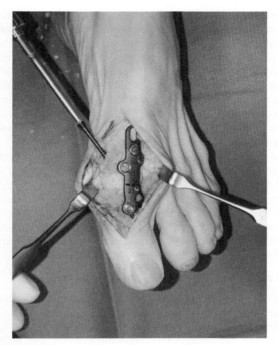

Fig. 6. Dorsal plating with lag screw.

conclusion, dorsal plate with concomitant lag screw is superior to crossed screws. The use of a locking plates compared to a nonlocking plate is associated with higher cost to the public without statistical improvement in union rates. However, patients with inflammatory arthropathy have shown higher fusion rates and shorter time to fusion with the use of precontoured locking plates.[28]

Postoperative Protocol

Mckeever allowed patients' heel weight-bearing in a cut out shoes after 4 days for 6 weeks.[7] Most investigators recommend similar protocols with use of a boot or postoperative rigid shoes when fixed with plate.[12,29,30] With screws fixation only, Brodsky and colleagues recommended 4 weeks of nonweight-bearing.[10] The investigators advocate for immediate heel weight-bearing followed by advancement to full weight-bearing in 4 weeks.

OUTCOMES

Brodsky and colleagues reported excellent pain relief following first MTP arthrodesis with an average pain score of 11 out of 100 at follow-up. Additionally, 36% of the patient population was completely pain free. Over 90% of patients could use stairs and walk more than 6 blocks without limitation, 98% returned to work. The return to sport ranged from 75% (jogging and tennis) to 92% (hiking). Forty-five percent could wear the shoes of their choice, while 47% preferred comfort shoes. Eight percent needed extra-depth shoes with custom orthoses. Only 64% could stand on tiptoes, while kneeling and picking up an object from the floor was reported at 94% and 98%, respectively.[10]

Satisfactory rates were also reported in other similar studies. In a study by DeSandis and colleagues, patient outcome data were reviewed. Short form health status survey (SF-36/12) improved from 65.7 to 81.2, and mean Foot and Ankle Outcomes Survey (FAOS) from 54.4 to 82.6. Eighty five percent of patients were satisfied or highly satisfied and 81% would undergo the same procedure again. The most common complaint among patient was the limitation in the height of heels. When evaluating the effect on age, 23% of younger patients reported limitation in daily and athletic activities which was similar to the older patients. The mean Visual Analogue Score score decreased from 6.1 on both group to 2.2 in the younger group and 2.9 in the older group. About 5% of patients reported a worsening in their functional outcomes.[29]

There is limited literature on long-term outcomes following first MTP arthrodesis.[12,30] Chraim and colleagues reported an average follow-up of 47.3 months (range 39–56 months) in 60 patients with 6.7% nonunion rate. Interestingly, there were no documented revisions for this, but 3.3% of patients underwent removal of hardware. Coughlin and Shurnas reported 34 cases of first MTP arthrodesis with a mean follow-up of 6.7 years. There were 2 cases of reoperation for hardware removals and 2 cases of painless fibrous nonunion. These results demonstrated satisfactory outcomes at nearly 7 year follow-up with low rate of reoperation.

Arthrodesis After Failed Joint-sparing or as Salvage Procedures

First MTP arthrodesis is widely accepted as the main salvage procedure after failed joint-sparing procedures.

Prior cheilectomy does not increase serious complication or fusion rate after conversion to first MTP arthrodesis.[31] Comparing primary first MTP arthrodesis to conversion first MTP arthrodesis after cheilectomy, Rajan and colleagues reported similar improvement in function between the 2 groups. On rare occasion, bone grafting is required after aggressive cheilectomy.[32] After Moberg osteotomy, optimal positioning of the toe could become challenging given the amount and location of prior bone excision.[33] There is limited literature about arthrodesis after interposition arthroplasty.

Myerson and colleagues reported outcomes in 24 patients who underwent first MTP arthrodesis after failed arthroplasty or Keller resection.[34] The defects were of at least 10 mm necessitating structural grafts to avoid medial column shortening in nearly all cases. The grafts were harvested from iliac crest, calcaneus, or resected metatarsal heads. The patients were all nonweight-bearing for 6 weeks following conversion. Reoperation rate was significant, with over half of the patients (7 out of 12) needing further surgery, including hardware removal due to irritation or prominence. The time to fusion averaged 6.9 months but with a wide variation of 3 to 18 months. Delayed union rate was high and occurred in 41.7% of cases. Patients requiring conversion from silicone implants, however, tended to achieve fusion more rapidly with an average time to union of 4.6 months. No patient was completely pain free, yet the majority still reported satisfactory results, with 25% achieving excellent outcomes and another 41.7% reporting good outcomes. Brodsky and colleagues reported similar outcome with no patient completely pain free and an average time to fusion of 3 to 4 months following conversion to first MTP arthrodesis.[35] After synthetic cartilage implant, Grimm and Irwin reported significant bone stock defects which required structural bone grafts.[36]

Both Myerson and colleagues and Brodsky and colleagues reported zero nonunion in patients treated with structural allografts, suggesting a potential benefit of allograft use in these conversion procedures.[34,35] Bei and colleagues reported a 90.9% fusion rate in a retrospective study in which dual plating (dorsal and medial) and allograft were used[37] (**Fig. 7**). In this study, 11 patients with bone defects for various etiology such as failed previous surgery or severe rheumatoid arthritis had an average of 11 ± 4.5 mm length restauration and average time to fusion of 10.7 ± 1 weeks. An extensive description of the double-plating procedure has been published by DeCarbo and colleagues.[38]

BIOMECHANICS AFTER FIRST METATARSOPHALANGEAL ARTHRODESIS

In a cadaveric study, Tan and colleagues measured the loss of flexor digitorum longus (FDL) excursion and lesser toe range of motion after first MTP arthrodesis. The release of the FDL at the knot of Henry improved function.[39] The investigators suggest further studies to investigate the benefits of this procedure on metatarsalgia after first MTP joint arthrodesis. A pedobarographic analysis showed an increased in maximal force value under both the first and second metatarsal head after fusion compared to the contralateral foot and a higher peak pressure under the first metatarsal head than under the second.[30] The contact surface was more balanced on the operative side between the first and second metatarsal head. The contralateral nonoperative foot showed increased contact surface value under the second metatarsal head.

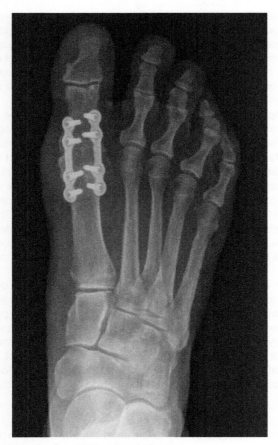

Fig. 7. Dual plating for the first MTP arthrodesis.

COMPLICATION AFTER FIRST METATARSOPHALANGEAL ARTHRODESIS

In recent literature, the first MTP arthrodesis fusion rates vary from 77% to 100%.[30] The largest series of 409 patients reported a nonunion rate of 8.6%, with 29.4% of the nonunion being symptomatic and requiring revision surgery.[40] Multiple variables were analyzed, and only preoperative hallux valgus was associated with higher nonunion rate. Weigelt and colleagues underlined the role of residual hallux valgus as a risk factor for nonunion. This large series was one of the only that didn't show a superiority of a dorsal plate construct over crossed screws.[41] A retrospective multicenter analysis of 794 patients who underwent first MTP arthrodesis with either crossed screws, dorsal plating with lag screw, or plate only reported an overall nonunion rate of 15.2% with 72.7% of these patients having a symptomatic nonunion.[42] Nonunion rate was 16.4% for crossed screws, 11.0% for a plate with an interfragmentary screw, and 21.2% for plate fixation only. Of note, flat cuts had a nonunion rate of 8.5% compared to 16.2% after preparation with convex and concave reamers.

Fitzgerald reported outcomes over a decade for 100 cases of first MTP arthrodesis.[43] The study reported that only 16 cases of malunions, which included 9 cases of pronation and 6 of insufficient valgus correction. In a more recent systematic review by Roukis , 2818 arthrodesis cases had a malunion rate of 6.1%. The majority (87.1%) of these malunions were characterized by sagittal malalignment with dorsal positioning of the hallux.[44] A review of 120 consecutive first MTP arthrodesis cases by Drittenbass and colleagues recorded a malunion rate of 9%. A majority of these malunions were related to insufficient extension and excessive valgus.[45] Despite the extensive literature on the first MTP arthrodesis, there is a scarcity of research specifically addressing malunion. When a malunion causes symptoms, corrective options such as opening or closing wedge osteotomies can be employed as salvage procedures to alleviate the discomfort.

Additional complications following the first MTP arthrodesis is the development of adjacent joint arthritis in the IP joint. In a series by Brodsky and colleagues, the degree of IP arthrosis as measured with the grading scale described by Fitzgerald demonstrated 68% of patients had stage I arthritis, 2% had stage II arthritis, and 17% had stage III arthritis.[10] No patient was noted to have stage IV disease in the IP joint. All patients denied having clinical symptoms of discomfort at the IP joint at the time of last follow-up.

Fitzgerald and colleagues reported 25% of patients had radiological IP joint arthritis 10 years after first MTP arthrodesis. Of these patients, 10% were symptomatic. IP joint arthrodesis following a prior first MTP joint arthrodesis has a recorded nonunion rate approaching 40%.[46] DeCarbo and colleagues report that fixation in excessive dorsiflexion of the first MTP leads to IP joint contracture and may lead to acceleration of arthrosis.[38]

Sesamoiditis is often associated with hallux rigidus.[47] Doty and colleagues found 74% of tibial sesamoids and 38% of fibular sesamoids with signs of articular erosions in 39 cadavers with concurrent hallux rigidus. Treatment of this problem is rarely discussed when performing the first MTP joint arthrodesis. Alshouli and colleagues reported satisfactory results after simultaneous first MTP arthrodesis and total sesamoidectomy.[48] In our experience, the routine sesamoidectomy is not necessary, and isolated cases with sesamoiditis treated with secondary sesamoidectomy present satisfactory outcome. These observations have also been reported by Tan and Lau.[49]

SUMMARY

In conclusion, the evolution of first MTP arthrodesis since its inception has been marked by a commitment to refining surgical techniques and expanding the understanding of hallux rigidus. From McKeever's pioneering work in the 1950s to contemporary practices, the procedure has remained a cornerstone for managing end-stage hallux rigidus, despite a burgeoning array of alternative treatments. The evidence underscores that while the first MTP arthrodesis can deliver substantial relief and restore function, particularly in patients with specific clinical profiles, it is not a one-size-fits-all remedy. The surgical community continues to grapple with the challenges of optimizing outcomes, such as the delicate balance between fusion and function, the nuances of joint preparation and fixation methods, and the management of complications and revisions. Nevertheless, the literature attests to the procedure's efficacy, offering a reliable option for those who have exhausted other treatments. Future endeavors in this field are anticipated to refine patient selection criteria further, improve surgical techniques, and enhance postoperative care, all aiming to provide tailored solutions that align with the etymologic roots of innovation—to make the first MTP joint "new again."

CLINICS CARE POINTS

- Immediate heel weight-bearing for 6 weeks, followed by full weight-bearing within 4 weeks is the most common postoperative protocol.
- Correct positioning of the arthrodesis is critical for the success of the surgery.
- Long-term outcomes are good, with a low number of revisions once fusion is achieved.
- Interphalangeal arthritis is a potential long-term complication.

DISCLOSURE

M.E. Easley is a consultant for Paragon 28 and Treace Medical. A.S. Acker and J. Liles have no commercial or financial conflicts of interest related to this work.

SUPPLEMENTARY DATA

Supplementary data related to this article can be found online at https://doi.org/10.1016/j.fcl.2024.02.008

REFERENCES

1. Senga Y, Nishimura A, Ito N, et al. Prevalence of and risk factors for hallux rigidus: a cross-sectional study in Japan. BMC Muscoskel Disord 2021;22(1):786.
2. Gould N, Schneider W, Ashikaga T. Epidemiological survey of foot problems in the continental United States: 1978-1979. Foot Ankle 1980;1(1):8–10.
3. Smith RW, Katchis SD, Ayson LC. Outcomes in hallux rigidus patients treated nonoperatively: a long-term follow-up study. Foot Ankle Int 2000;21(11):906–13.
4. Shariff R, Myerson MS. The Use of Osteotomy in the Management of Hallux Rigidus. Foot Ankle Clin 2015;20(3):493–502.
5. Kon Kam King C, Loh Sy J, Zheng Q, et al. Comprehensive Review of Non-Operative Management of Hallux Rigidus. Cureus 2017;9(1):e987.
6. Clutton H. The treatment of hallux valgus. St Thomas Rep 1894;22:1–12.
7. McKeever DC. Arthrodesis of the first metatarsophalangeal joint for hallux valgus, hallux rigidus, and metatarsus primus varus. J Bone Joint Surg Am 1952;34-A(1):129–34.

8. Thompson FR, Mcelvenny RT. Arthrodesis of the first metatarsophalangeal joint. JBJS 1940;22(3):555–8.

9. Fuhrmann RA. First metatarsophalangeal arthrodesis for hallux rigidus. Foot Ankle Clin 2011;16(1):1–12.

10. Brodsky JW, Passmore RN, Pollo FE, et al. Functional outcome of arthrodesis of the first metatarsophalangeal joint using parallel screw fixation. Foot Ankle Int 2005;26(2):140–6.

11. Lacoste KL, Andrews NA, Ray J, et al. First Metatarsophalangeal Joint Arthrodesis: A Narrative Review of Fixation Constructs and Their Evolution. Cureus 2021;13(4):e14458.

12. Coughlin MJ, Shurnas PS. Hallux rigidus. Grading and long-term results of operative treatment. J Bone Joint Surg Am 2003;85(11):2072–88.

13. Hodel S, Viehofer A, Wirth S. Minimally invasive arthrodesis of the first metatarsophalangeal joint: A systematic literature review. Foot Ankle Surg 2020;26(6):601–6.

14. Edwards WH. Avascular necrosis of the first metatarsal head. Foot Ankle Clin 2005;10(1):117–27.

15. de Prado M, Ripoll P-L and Golanó P. Minimally Invasive Management of Hallux Rigidus, In: Maffulli N. and Easley M., *Minimally invasive surgery of the foot and ankle*, 2011, London: Springer London, 75–87.

16. Wilson JN. Cone arthrodesis of the first metatarso-phalangeal joint. The Journal of Bone & Joint Surgery British 1967;49-B(1):98–101.

17. Ho B, Baumhauer J. Hallux rigidus. EFORT Open Rev 2017;2(1):13–20.

18. Galois L, Hemmer J, Ray V, et al. Surgical options for hallux rigidus: state of the art and review of the literature. Eur J Orthop Surg Traumatol 2020;30(1):57–65.

19. Lambrinudi C. Metatarsus Primus Elevatus. Proc R Soc Med 1938;31(11):1273.

20. Politi J, John H, Njus G, et al. First metatarsal-phalangeal joint arthrodesis: a biomechanical assessment of stability. Foot Ankle Int 2003;24(4):332–7.

21. Lewis JT, Hanselman AE, Lalli TA, et al. Effect of Dorsal Plate Positioning on Dorsiflexion Angle in Arthrodesis of the First Metatarsophalangeal Joint: A Cadaveric Study. Foot Ankle Int 2014;35(8):802–8.

22. Haimes MA, Roberts MS, Bougioukas L, et al. Analysis of the Costs and Complications of First Metatarsophalangeal Joint Arthrodesis Comparing Locked and Non-locked Plate Fixation Constructs. J Am Acad Orthop Surg 2023;31(21):e1012–20.

23. Claassen L, Plaass C, Pastor MF, et al. First Metatarsophalangeal Joint Arthrodesis: A Retrospective Comparison of Crossed-screws, Locking and Non-Locking Plate Fixation with Lag Screw. Arch Bone Jt Surg 2017;5(4):221–5.

24. Hunt KJ, Ellington JK, Anderson RB, et al. Locked versus nonlocked plate fixation for hallux MTP arthrodesis. Foot Ankle Int 2011;32(7):704–9.

25. Doty J, Coughlin M, Hirose C, et al. Hallux metatarsophalangeal joint arthrodesis with a hybrid locking plate and a plantar neutralization screw: a prospective study. Foot Ankle Int 2013;34(11):1535–40.

26. Balu AR, Baumann AN, Tsang T, et al. Evaluating the Biomechanical Integrity of Various Constructs Utilized for First Metatarsophalangeal Joint Arthrodesis: A Systematic Review. Materials 2023;(19):16.

27. Schafer KA, Baldini T, Hamati M, et al. Two Orthogonal Nitinol Staples and Combined Nitinol Staple-Screw Constructs for a First Metatarsophalangeal Joint Arthrodesis: A Biomechanical Cadaver Study. Foot Ankle Int 2022;43(11):1493–500.

28. Mayer SA, Zelenski NA, DeOrio JK, et al. A comparison of nonlocking semitubular plates and precontoured locking plates for first metatarsophalangeal joint arthrodesis. Foot Ankle Int 2014;35(5):438–44.
29. DeSandis B, Pino A, Levine DS, et al. Functional Outcomes Following First Metatarsophalangeal Arthrodesis. Foot Ankle Int 2016;37(7):715–21.
30. Chraim M, Bock P, Alrabai HM, et al. Long-term outcome of first metatarsophalangeal joint fusion in the treatment of severe hallux rigidus. Int Orthop 2016;40(11): 2401–8.
31. Rajan L, Kim J, An T, et al. Effect of Prior Cheilectomy on Outcomes of First Metatarsophalangeal Joint Fusion for Treatment of Hallux Rigidus. Foot Ankle Orthop 2022;7(3). 24730114221119740.
32. Tomlinson M. Pain after cheilectomy of the first metatarsophalangeal joint: diagnosis and management. Foot Ankle Clin 2014;19(3):349–60.
33. O'Malley MJ, Basran HS, Gu Y, et al. Treatment of advanced stages of hallux rigidus with cheilectomy and phalangeal osteotomy. J Bone Joint Surg Am 2013; 95(7):606–10.
34. Myerson MS, Schon LC, McGuigan FX, et al. Result of arthrodesis of the hallux metatarsophalangeal joint using bone graft for restoration of length. Foot Ankle Int 2000;21(4):297–306.
35. Brodsky JW, Ptaszek AJ, Morris SG. Salvage first MTP arthrodesis utilizing ICBG: clinical evaluation and outcome. Foot Ankle Int 2000;21(4):290–6.
36. Grimm MPD, Irwin TA. Complications of Hallux Rigidus Surgery. Foot Ankle Clin 2022;27(2):253–69.
37. Bei C, Gross CE, Adams S, et al. Dual plating with bone block arthrodesis of the first metatarsophalangeal joint: A clinical retrospective review. Foot Ankle Surg 2015;21(4):235–9.
38. DeCarbo WT, Dayton P, Smith WB, et al. Triplanar Correction for First Metatarsophalangeal Fusion. J Foot Ankle Surg 2021;60(5):1044–7.
39. Tan CY, Bin Mohd Fadil MF. Biomechanical consequences of first metatarsaophalangeal joint arthrodesis on flexor digitorum longus function: A cadaveric study. J Orthop Surg 2019;27(1). 2309499019826325.
40. Kannan S, Bennett A, Chong HH, et al. A Multicenter Retrospective Cohort Study of First Metatarsophalangeal Joint Arthrodesis. J Foot Ankle Surg 2021;60(3): 436–9.
41. Weigelt L, Redfern J, Heyes GJ, et al. Risk Factors for Nonunion After First Metatarsophalangeal Joint Arthrodesis With a Dorsal Locking Plate and Compression Screw Construct: Correction of Hallux Valgus Is Key. J Foot Ankle Surg 2021; 60(6):1179–83.
42. Fussenich W, Seeber GH, van Raaij TM, et al. Factors Associated With Nonunion in Arthrodesis of the First Metatarsophalangeal Joint: A Multicenter Retrospective Cohort Study. Foot Ankle Int 2023;44(6):508–15.
43. Fitzgerald JA. A review of long-term results of arthrodesis of the first metatarsophalangeal joint. J Bone Joint Surg Br 1969;51(3):488–93.
44. Roukis TS. Nonunion after arthrodesis of the first metatarsal-phalangeal joint: a systematic review. J Foot Ankle Surg 2011;50(6):710–3.
45. Drittenbass L, Kutaish H, Chin LV, et al. Why and How Often Is Revision Surgery Necessary after First Metatarsophalangeal Joint Arthrodeses? A Cohort of 120 Consecutive Cases. Open J Orthoped 2021;11(08):221–32.
46. Brodsky JW, Zide JR, Kim KES, et al. Arthrodesis of Ipsilateral Hallux Metatarsophalangeal and Interphalangeal Joints. Foot Ankle Orthop 2021;6(1). 2473011 420983815.

47. Doty JF, Coughlin MJ, Schutt S, et al. Articular chondral damage of the first metatarsal head and sesamoids: analysis of cadaver hallux valgus. Foot Ankle Int 2013;34(8):1090–6.
48. Alshouli MT, Lin A, Kadakia AR. Simultaneous first metatarsophalangeal joint arthrodesis and sesamoidectomy with a single dorsomedial incision. Foot Ankle Spec 2014;7(5):403–8.
49. Tan J, Lau JT. Metatarso-sesamoid osteoarthritis as a cause of pain after first metatarsophalangeal joint fusion: case report. Foot Ankle Int 2011;32(8):822–5.

The Philosophy of Surgical Success and Outcomes of Cartiva Versus Fusion

Solangel Rodriguez-Materon, MD, Gregory P. Guyton, MD*

KEYWORDS

- Synthetic cartilage implant • Noninferiority trial • Statistical analysis • Hallux rigidus
- Arthrodesis

KEY POINTS

- Noninferiority study design requires investigator assumptions to arrive at a binary definition of success and the level of rigor of the study.
- Surgical decision-making is more nuanced and reflects a surgical philosophy that may not match that of a noninferiority study.
- Careful consideration of study design, especially of criteria for success, is essential for surgical decision-making.
- Residual pain is a factor that warrants special attention by the surgeon for appropriate patient guidance and surgical decision- making.

WHAT IS A NONINFERIORITY TRIAL?

Noninferiority clinical trial design is used when a superiority trial is not feasible or when an existing treatment is known to be effective. Initially, noninferiority trials were used in pharmaceutical research where it would be unethical to withhold a known effective treatment in treating a serious disease like acquired immunodeficiency syndrome(AIDS) or cancer. Noninferiority trial design began to be used for other treatments, including surgery, to address regulatory requirements for new procedures or devices. In addition to allowing all patients to receive some form of effective treatment, noninferiority trials also typically require fewer participants than superiority trials.

Surgical noninferiority trials often rely upon a definition of surgical success supplied by the investigators that incorporates their own philosophies of care. A noninferiority trial might find that a new treatment is less effective in 1 area of concern than a known treatment but offers an advantage in another area considered desirable by surgeons or patients. One common design typically used for regulatory approval by the Food

Department of Orthopaedic Surgery, MedStar Union Memorial Hospital, 3333 North Calvert Street, Suite 400, Baltimore, MD 21218, USA
* Corresponding author.
E-mail address: gpguyton@gmail.com

Foot Ankle Clin N Am 29 (2024) 521–527
https://doi.org/10.1016/j.fcl.2023.12.001
1083-7515/24/© 2023 Elsevier Inc. All rights reserved.

and Drug Administration (FDA) relies upon satisfying a checklist composed of the absence of safety events, improvement on a patient-reported outcome, and measurable objective functional criteria.

In addition to the classic parameters of significance (α) and power (β), noninferiority trials have a third defining parameter: the noninferiority margin (M). This margin is the degree to which the new treatment may yield worse results than the existing treatment and still be considered "noninferior." In studies using a continuous variable such as a patient-reported outcome scale, the margin is typically set to equal the minimal clinically important difference (MCID) of that scale. If, as in most surgical trials, a categorical outcome of success or failure is used as the primary outcome variable, the noninferiority margin is arbitrary and must be set by consensus. By convention, a noninferiority margin of 10% has been used by the FDA for most orthopedic pivotal trials, though the investigators can argue for a higher margin based on the perceived strength of a known benefit of the new treatment. A larger noninferiority margin increases the chances that the new treatment will be found noninferior to the existing treatment.

The primary outcome for a noninferiority trial can be difficult to understand. For a study with a 5% statistical significance, the 95% confidence interval for the difference in outcomes between the original treatment and the new treatment is used. The lower boundary of that interval is then compared to the predetermined noninferiority margin. If both treatments yield equal outcomes, the difference between them will be 0. Therefore, if the lower boundary of the 95% CI for that difference is less than the noninferiority margin, the new treatment is demonstrated to be "noninferior" (**Fig. 1**).

This convention leads to another arbitrary choice in study design. Since only the lower boundary of the 95% CI for the differences of outcomes is used, some investigators have chosen to use a *1-sided* confidence interval that excludes 5% of the possible outcomes from only 1 side of the scale. In contrast, a conventional *2-sided* confidence interval excludes 2.5% of the possible outcomes from each end of the scale. Either technique can be defended, and both have appeared in the orthopedic

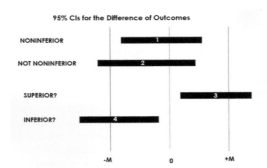

Fig. 1. Possible outcomes of a noninferiority trial. The difference of outcomes with a 2-sided 95% CI is shown for 4 possible conditions: (1) A trial in which the lower bound of the 95% CI is above the noninferiority margin. This outcome is "noninferior."(2) A trial in which the lower bound of the 95% CI is below the noninferiority margin. This outcome is "not noninferior."(3) A trial in which the entire 95% confidence interval is below 0. This demonstrates "inferiority" of the new treatment. (4) A trial in which the entire 95% CI is above 0. This demonstrates superiority of the new treatment. It should be noted that noninferiority trials are not typically powered to demonstrate superiority and inferiority, and these outcomes are not usually supported in the data.

literature. It is very important to note, however, that the lower boundary of a 1-sided 95% CI is identical to that of a 90% 2-sided interval. Designs that use a 1-sided interval are substantially less rigorous than those that use 2-sided intervals.

THE FDA PIVOTAL TRIAL FOR CARTIVA: THE MOTION STUDY

The MOTION study is a well-known multicenter, unblinded, randomized controlled noninferiority trial that found Cartiva, a novel motion-preserving cylindrical polyvinyl first metatarsophalangeal (MTP) implant, noninferior to arthrodesis for treatment of first metatarsophalangeal joint degeneration.[1] It was designed with a 2:1 randomization, but many patients chose to crossover to the motion-preserving Cartiva implant. The MOTION trial ultimately included 130 patients in the Cartiva group and 50 patients in the arthrodesis group for final analysis.

MOTION TRIAL METHODS

The study utilized a checklist of standards to generate a categorical success/failure outcome for each participant (**Table 1**).[2] The primary outcome variable was the difference in the success–failure proportion for the implant compared with the standard treatment of MTP arthrodesis. The study was a 1-sided 95% CI, and a noninferiority margin of −15% was used.[3] As noted earlier, the combination of a 1-sided 95% CI and a −15% noninferiority margin was less rigorous than typically used by the FDA and matched the least rigorous trial to appear in the orthopedic literature to date.[2] In internal FDA documents, the trial designers justified the use of a less rigorous margin by their perception that a faster return to function would occur and that preservation of MTP motion was very desirable.[4]

RESULTS OF THE MOTION TRIAL

The MOTION trial found Cartiva to be noninferior to arthrodesis using its preestablished criteria for success. The lower boundary of a 1-sided 95% confidence interval for this difference of the proportions of success for Cartiva versus arthrodesis was 10.4%. Had a 2-sided confidence interval been used, the lower boundary would

Table 1	
Criteria for surgical success in the MOTION trial[2,4]	
Criterion	**Description**
Pain	Improvement (decrease) from baseline in visual analog scale (VAS) Pain of ≥30% at 24 mo
Function	Maintenance of function from baseline in the foot and ankle ability measure (FAAM) Activities of Daily living (ADL) score at 24 mo (inclusive of decrease <8)
Safety	Freedom from major complications[a] and subsequent secondary surgical interventions through 24 mo
Radiographic	Absence of predetermined radiographic failure criteria including nonunion in the case of arthrodesis and component migration in the case of the Cartiva implant.

[a] Major complications were defined from radiographic findings and were assessed by an independent radiographic reviewer. These included absence of device displacement, device fragmentation, and avascular necrosis in the Cartiva group and the absence of malunion, non-union, and hardware fractures in the fusion group. Painless pseudoarthrosis and isolated hardware removal were considered to represent failure in the fusion group.

have been −13.0%. Both of these values were below the margin typically used by the FDA for orthopedic devices, but above the more permissive margin chosen in the trial design.

In addition to the choice of margin and type of confidence interval, the components of the checklist to define success warrant additional attention.

Secondary Surgeries

For both Cartiva and arthrodesis, adverse events and subsequent surgeries occurred. A total of 14 (9.2%) Cartiva patients and 6 (12%) fusion patients had secondary surgery. Ten Cartiva implants were converted to fusion, one patient underwent a Moberg osteotomy, and one had repositioning of the implant. Three arthrodesis patients underwent revision fusion for nonunion. Additionally, several smaller procedures occurred. One Cartiva patient underwent a scar release and 3 arthrodesis patients underwent hardware removal. Of these, one of the patients with hardware removal underwent subsequent revision fusion.

The trial treated all secondary surgical events as categorical failures, equating more minor hardware removal with the major procedure of revision fusion. Alternatively, it may be reasonable to consider only major revisions or bony surgeries as failures while considering simple hardware removal or scar revision as successes if symptoms were alleviated. If this approach is taken, the lower boundary of the 95% CI for the difference of proportions changes to − 15.1%, a value below the −15% margin that indicates Cartiva does not meet the threshold for noninferiority to fusion.

X-ray Interpretation

The reported overall radiographic success rate was 100% for the Cartiva group and 90% for the fusion group.[4] Radiographic anomalies were counted as failure regardless of whether they were associated with pain. Three patients in the arthrodesis group were counted as radiographic failures despite the absence of pain (1 broken hardware and 2 pseudoarthrosis).[2]

Alternatively, it may be reasonable to consider a painless outcome to be a success regardless of the radiographic appearance, particularly when an inadvertent but painless pseudarthrosis from attempted fusion is compared to a procedure that is itself designed to create just such a painless pseudarthrosis. If the 3 arthrodesis patients with painless radiographic anomalies are reclassified as successes, the lower boundary of the 95% CI for the difference of proportions changes to −15.9%, a value below the −15% margin that indicates Cartiva does not meet the threshold for noninferiority to fusion.

Pain Threshold Modeling Versus Percentage Improvement

A statistically and clinically significant reduction in pain was reported in nearly 89% of the Cartiva population and in 97% of the fusion population for those subjects reaching the 24-month endpoint without any subsequent secondary surgical interventions.[4] The trial used a 30% improvement of visual analog scale (VAS) pain score as a criterion for success, a value appropriately greater than those commonly accepted for MCID for VAS pain supported by the literature.[5,6]

An alternative and increasingly used paradigm is that of the Patient Acceptable Symptomatic State (PASS) score. This model requires that a patient reach a threshold of diminished symptoms that are considered "acceptable" rather than simply achieving some percentage of improvement. It can be succinctly stated as "it is more important to feel good than to feel better." If a VAS pain threshold of 30, a reasonable and permissive PASS threshold, is used as the criterion for success in the MOTION study, 6 Cartiva patients previously considered successes would be recategorized as failures. In other words, although their pain improved somewhat, they still had very significant symptoms at the end of the trial. No arthrodesis patients had similar parameters. As shown in **Fig. 2**, the positive standard error for pain in the Cartiva group remained above a VAS pain threshold of 30 through 24 months, while that for arthrodesis did not.[2]

If a VAS pain threshold of 30 rather than a 30% reduction in VAS pain is used as the criterion for success, the lower boundary of the 1-sided 95% CI for the difference of proportions changes to −15.8%, a value below the −15% margin that indicates Cartiva does not meet the threshold for noninferiority to fusion.

POST-MARKET EXPERIENCE WITH CARTIVA

The positive findings for Cartiva in the MOTION trial have not been universally replicated in subsequent Level IV retrospective studies. A retrospective chart review of 60 patients with implantation of Cartiva and mean follow-up of 18.5 months (range 12–30 months) found that only 14% of patients were very satisfied, 20% neutral, 11% unsatisfied, and 27% very unsatisfied with their outcome. These investigators noted a 20% reoperation rate, which included an 8% rate of conversion to arthrodesis and up to 52% of patients with postoperative corticosteroid injection due to continued discomfort.[7]

In a retrospective review of 103 patients who underwent first MTP hemiarthroplasty with Cartiva with average follow-up of 26.2 months, 50.5% of the patients had a concurrent Moberg proximal phalanx osteotomy. Mean physical function and pain scores improved significantly preoperatively to postoperatively, but postoperative pain scores were significantly higher for patients who had undergone a prior procedure of the first MTP and significantly lower for patients who underwent concurrent Moberg osteotomy. There were only 2 revision procedures in the first 2 years postoperatively.[8] A later study from the same institution compared 72 patients who underwent cheilectomy and Moberg osteotomy plus Cartiva and 94 patients with the same procedures without Cartiva. At 1 to 2 years of follow-up, both groups demonstrated significant improvement in all Patient-Reported Outcomes Measurement Information System (PROMIS) domains scores. However, the group without Cartiva had significantly higher postoperative physical function and significantly lower pain intensity scores with fewer postoperative complications.[9]

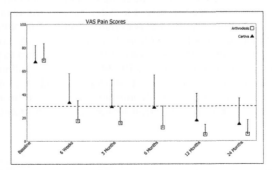

Fig. 2. Visual analog scale (VAS) pain scores over time in the motion study.[2] Dotted line, 30-mm VAS pain threshold value. (Reproduced with permission from Guyton GP, *Philosophies of Surgical Care are Embedded in Outcome Studies: An Illustrative Reanalysis of the Cartiva MOTION Trial. Foot Ankle Int* 2022; 43(10) 1364-369.)

A retrospective chart review of 59 feet treated with Cartiva with average follow-up of 18.9 months reported significant improvement from preoperatively to most recent follow-up for the Foot and Ankle Ability Measure (FAAM) Activities of Daily Living (ADL) (71.0 vs 88.2 points), FAAM Sports (44.6 vs 72.0 points), and VAS (49.4 vs 31.0) (P<.01). Ten patients (18.5%) required revision surgery. Of those, 7 patients were revised to an arthrodesis, 1 metal hemiarthroplasty, and 2 implants were removed because of infection.[10]

A small case series reported radiological outcomes of 11 patients who underwent treatment with Cartiva with mean follow-up of 20.9 months. Implant subsidence was seen in 60% of the cases at 4 weeks after surgery and 90% at final follow-up. A total of 50% of patients showed radiologic lucency around the implant, 40% had erosion of the proximal phalanx of the great toe, and 36% reported no improvement at final follow-up and were considered as treatment failures. Of the 11 patients, 3 required revision surgery.[11]

A large single-surgeon series retrospective review of 146 patients who underwent Cartiva treatment for hallux rigidus with a minimum 6-month follow-up (mean 14.5 months) found that patients experienced significant improvement in VAS and hallux dorsiflexion postoperatively.[12] There were 22 (15.1%) complications including implant subsidence (10.3%), deep infection (4.1%), and hypertrophic ossification (0.7%). Revision surgeries were required in X (12.3%) of patients at an average of 9.4 months postoperatively. The 1-year and 2-year survival to arthrodesis (n = 9) were 95.9% and 86.3%, respectively.

SURGICAL PHILOSOPHY AND THE CARTIVA IMPLANT

Noninferiority studies in surgery are, by their very nature, reductionist. They use multiple variables to generate a yes or no answer about the new device being tested. Whereas a binary outcome is appropriate for a regulatory agency such as the FDA, the clinical situation is more nuanced. It is critical to understand the underlying philosophies and choices that go into trial design when a surgeon is recommending a new device. In the case of Cartiva, any of 3 reasonable alternative means of defining surgical success would have altered the final outcome of the MOTION trial. Additionally, using a more rigorous noninferiority margin rather than adding an additional cushion based upon the argument that motion alone had extra inherent value would have also led to failure of the trial to demonstrate noninferiority.

The MOTION trial remains a significant accomplishment, but interpreting its results at the level of an individual patient requires looking beyond the overall noninferiority outcome and into the secondary results. A construction worker simply interested in reliable pain relief should clearly be offered a fusion, and a professional yoga instructor who is willing to risk a less reliable outcome with regard to pain to preserve toe motion may be a candidate for Cartiva. The MOTION trial continues to serve as a model both because it was extensive and remarkably well-documented, but also because its outcomes can be so variably interpreted based upon the philosophies of the individual surgeon and patient. That lesson, so vividly demonstrated in this case, is universal.

CLINICS CARE POINTS

- Physician philosophies of care and patient expectations are not universal, and they may not match those reflected in even the most carefully designed investigations.

- Careful patient selection and choice of surgical procedures are crucial for successful treatment.
- If a motion-sparing technique is used over arthrodesis, discussion of possible complications, conversion to fusion, and pain relief expectations is critical.

DISCLOSURE

The authors declare no potential conflicts of interest with respect to the research, authorship, and/or publication of this article. ICMJE forms for all authors are available online. No disclosures related to this article.

REFERENCES

1. Baumhauer JF, Singh D, Glazebrook M, et al. Prospective, randomized, multi-centered clinical trial assessing safety and efficacy of a synthetic cartilage implant versus first metatarsophalangeal arthrodesis in advanced hallux rigidus. Foot Ankle Int 2016;37(5):457–69.
2. Guyton GP. Philosophies of surgical care are embedded in outcome studies: an illustrative reanalysis of the Cartiva MOTION trial. Foot Ankle Int 2022;43(10): 1364–9. Epub 20220818.
3. Guyton GP. Standards for noninferiority trials in orthopaedic surgery would be arbitrary: it's time we had some. J Bone Joint Surg Am 2021;103(17):e69. Epub 2021/04/02.
4. U.S. Food & Drug Administration. FDA Executive Summary: Cartiva Synthetic Cartilage Implant. Available at: https://www.fda.gov/media/96916/download. Accessed September 8, 2023. 2016.
5. Olsen MF, Bjerre E, Hansen MD, et al. Minimum clinically important differences in chronic pain vary considerably by baseline pain and methodological factors: systematic review of empirical studies. J Clin Epidemiol 2018;101:87–106 e2. Epub 2018/05/25.
6. Olsen MF, Bjerre E, Hansen MD, et al. Pain relief that matters to patients: systematic review of empirical studies assessing the minimum clinically important difference in acute pain. BMC Med 2017;15(1):35. Epub 2017/02/22.
7. Cassinelli SJ, Chen S, Charlton TP, et al. Early outcomes and complications of synthetic cartilage implant for treatment of hallux rigidus in the United States. Foot Ankle Int 2019;40(10):1140–8. Epub 2019/06/15.
8. Eble SK, Hansen OB, Chrea B, et al. Clinical outcomes of the polyvinyl alcohol (PVA) hydrogel implant for hallux rigidus. Foot Ankle Int 2020;41(9):1056–64. Epub 20200710.
9. Chrea B, Eble SK, Day J, et al. Comparison between polyvinyl alcohol implant and cheilectomy With Moberg osteotomy for hallux rigidus. Foot Ankle Int 2020;41(9):1031–40. Epub 2020/07/30.
10. Engasser WM, Coetzee JC, Ebeling PB, et al. Patient-reported outcomes and early complications after synthetic cartilage device implantation. Foot Ankle Orthop 2020;5(3). 2473011420930691. Epub 20200806.
11. Shimozono Y, Hurley ET, Kennedy JG. Early failures of polyvinyl alcohol hydrogel implant for the treatment of hallux rigidus. Foot Ankle Int 2021;42(3):340–6. Epub 2020/10/13.
12. Fletcher AN, Chopra A, Madi NS, et al. Polyvinyl alcohol hydrogel hemiarthroplasty of first metatarsophalangeal joint hallux rigidus: single surgeon five-year experience. Foot Ankle Orthop 2022;7(4).

DISCLOSURE

The authors declare no conflicts of interest with respect to the publication of this article.

REFERENCES

1.

2.

3.

4.

5.

6.

7.

8.

9.

10.

11.

12.

Effect of Prior Cheilectomy on Outcomes of First Metatarsophalangeal Joint Fusion

Rami Mizher, MD, Lavan Rajan, MD, Scott J. Ellis, MD*

KEYWORDS

- Hallux rigidus • Cheilectomy • First MTP fusion • Conversion arthrodesis

KEY POINTS

- Cheilectomy is a joint-preserving procedure effective for treating various stages of hallux rigidus.
- Conversion to metatarsophalangeal (MTP) joint fusion may be required if cheilectomy fails or arthritis progresses.
- Patients with a history of cheilectomy demonstrate comparable clinical improvement after MTP joint fusion to those without prior surgical history.
- Despite showing comparable clinical benefit after MTP fusion, patients with a history of cheilectomy demonstrate worse preoperative and postoperative function.

INTRODUCTION

In the evolving practice of foot and ankle surgery, the management and treatment of hallux rigidus remains a contentious topic with no consensus on a single best approach. Among the variety of treatment options available, the 2 procedures that are most widely performed include cheilectomy and first metatarsophalangeal (MTP) joint arthrodesis.

Cheilectomy, a joint-preserving procedure, is commonly performed to alleviate pain and restore some functional range of motion, often aided by a proximal phalangeal dorsiflexion osteotomy (Moberg osteotomy). However, first MTP joint arthrodesis involves the permanent fixation of the joint to eliminate pain and improve stability, although at the price of sacrificing motion. Despite their differences, both procedures have proven their efficacy in treating hallux rigidus, with varying degrees of success based on patient factors, expectations, and disease stage.

With an increasing number of patients undergoing cheilectomy in the hope of preventing or delaying joint fusion, a pertinent question arises: How does the history of

Foot and Ankle Department, Weill Cornell Medical College, Hospital for Special Surgery, New York, USA
* Corresponding author, The East River Professional Building 523, East 72nd St (5th Floor), between York and the East River.
E-mail address: elliss@hss.edu

Foot Ankle Clin N Am 29 (2024) 529–540
https://doi.org/10.1016/j.fcl.2023.10.005
1083-7515/24/© 2023 Elsevier Inc. All rights reserved.

cheilectomy affect the outcomes of first MTP joint fusion? This article will explore the relationship between the 2 procedures and aims to shed light on the implications of prior cheilectomy on the clinical outcomes of first MTP joint fusion.

NATURE OF THE PROBLEM

When deliberating between treatment options for arthritic conditions, orthopedic surgeons are almost always faced with a dilemma—the tradeoff between native joint function and pain. Approaching hallux rigidus is no different: should clinicians prioritize joint preservation and thereby maintain function at the risk of persistent pain and progression of arthritis? Alternatively, would it be more judicious to opt for a definitive option by addressing the root pathologic condition and fusing the joint at the expense of compromising function? Emerging research has provided more insight into the implications of prior cheilectomy on outcomes of first MTP joint arthrodesis, underscoring the viability of this approach in clinical practice.

CHEILECTOMY

Cheilectomy refers to the ostectomy of the distal portion of the articular surface of the first metatarsal head as well as any dorsal osteophytes on the metatarsal head or proximal phalanx (**Fig. 1**A). Commonly, this involves the resection of up to a third of the degenerated articular surface.[1] Traditionally, a cheilectomy has been recommended for initial stages of hallux rigidus with the goal of relieving the pain caused by impingement of the dorsal osteophytes.[1–3] Contemporary evidence, however, has

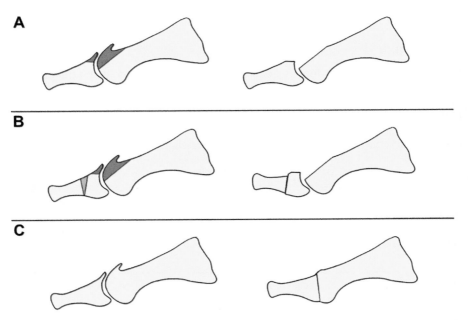

Fig. 1. Sagittal diagrams of the first MT joint depicting cheilectomy, cheilectomy with Moberg osteotomy, and MTP fusion. (*A*) The changes involved in cheilectomy, labeled in red. (*B*) The changes involved in cheilectomy (red) and Moberg osteotomy (blue). (*C*) The changes involved in MTP joint fusion using flat cuts (rather than cup and cone reamers), with the resultant proximal phalanx being set with 15° of dorsiflexion relative to the first metatarsal.

demonstrated the success of cheilectomy for more advanced stages of hallux rigidus.[4] Consequently, an increasing number of surgeons are opting for a cheilectomy as a primary intervention.

Although cheilectomy alone may improve the range of motion of the first MTP joint intraoperatively, postoperative clinical range of motion noticed by the patient may only be slightly improved. Studies have shown that although the intraoperative range of motion was noted to reach 80° to 90° of dorsiflexion, actual postoperative range of motion has been reported to be a maximum of 39°.[1,5–7] The functional gain in dorsiflexion is most noticeable when a cheilectomy is augmented by a proximal phalanx dorsal closing wedge osteotomy (Moberg osteotomy), which shifts the arc toward more dorsiflexion at the expense of plantarflexion. Nevertheless, cheilectomy is a highly successful joint-preserving technique that maintains the function and range of motion of the first MTP joint.

CHEILECTOMY WITH MOBERG OSTEOTOMY

A proximal phalanx dorsal closing wedge osteotomy, colloquially referred to as a Moberg osteotomy, is commonly performed in tandem with a cheilectomy (see **Fig. 1**B). Although the cheilectomy is primarily designed to alleviate the dorsal bony impingement, the Moberg osteotomy orients the proximal phalanx more dorsally, enhancing dorsiflexion and resulting in an arc of motion that is more clinically helpful to the patient.[8] Studies have demonstrated that combining a Moberg osteotomy with a cheilectomy can achieve a postoperative range of motion nearing 60° of dorsiflexion, markedly superior to the outcomes from a standalone cheilectomy.[4,9] When performed concomitantly, these procedures offer promising long-term results, even in advanced stages of hallux rigidus. Therefore, this combined intervention has gained traction as a primary therapy for patients, even those with advanced degeneration, who wish to preserve the integrity of their first MTP joint while seeking pain relief.

FIRST METATARSOPHALANGEAL JOINT ARTHRODESIS

Fusion of the first MTP joint is a definitive procedure aimed at definitively eliminating the source of the pain associated with hallux rigidus. It is more commonly performed for advanced arthritic stages and may be considered as a primary treatment strategy, foregoing preliminary attempts at cheilectomy if the probability of failure is likely to be high.[10] However, because this technique fuses the MTP joint, it will lead to more pronounced functional limitations, especially with activities involving substantial dorsiflexion (see **Fig. 1**C). This limitation is of a particular concern for patients with high activity levels, professionals such as dancers—most notably ballerinas—and individuals who prefer wearing high-heeled footwear, among others.[11,12] However, studies have shown that 96% of patients were satisfied with their return to sport after MTP fusion, indicating a positive prognosis for most activities after arthrodesis.[13]

Of course, there are specific scenarios where a primary first MTP fusion might be the most suitable intervention. As previously mentioned, patients presenting with advanced arthritis, wherein a cheilectomy might offer limited therapeutic improvement, could potentially benefit more from a fusion as a primary intervention. This approach can obviate an intermediary procedure with a foreseeable unfavorable outcome. Additionally, primary fusion is the preferred procedure in patients with hallux rigidus caused by rheumatoid arthritis in addition to those with coexisting hallux valgus or hallux varus because the abnormal bone alignment is more successfully addressed by a fusion rather than joint-conserving procedures with a high failure rate.[14,15] The option of a primary fusion becomes even more pertinent in patients with suboptimal bone stock or compromised bone quality. These could be patients with coexisting metabolic bone disorders such as osteoporosis, or those with diabetes or a history of chronic steroid use, both of which are known to degrade bone quality and can lead to osteopenia.[16,17] Given the inherently elevated risks of malunion, nonunion, and other associated complications in these patients even during a primary fusion, introducing a preliminary surgery, which could further deplete bone stock or alter bone quality, might only amplify the risks should a subsequent fusion become necessary.

THEORETICAL ISSUES OF PERFORMING CHEILECTOMY BEFORE FUSION

Although it is sensible to start with joint-preserving surgical techniques such as cheilectomy, to treat hallux rigidus, this does come with foreseeable risks that could affect subsequent joint fusion.

Decreased Bone Stock

As a cheilectomy involves resecting a segment of the degenerated articular surface, it can reduce the bone volume present at the metatarsal head, which is essential for successful fusion.[18] Osseous fusion depends on a variety of factors, both at the local mechanical and physiologic levels.[10,19,20] Therefore, any alteration to the osseous interface, the foundation for proper bridging and fusion, can affect the likelihood of achieving a successful union.[21]

Progression of Arthritis

Since cheilectomy is primarily performed for symptomatic pain relief rather than addressing the underlying pathologic condition, arthritic changes could continue to progress, risking increased joint degeneration. In fact, a study by Easley and colleagues showed that 43% of patients who experienced recurrence of the dorsal osteophyte after cheilectomy were predominantly symptomatic with pain at the midrange of motion, indicating the recurrence is largely due to progression of arthritis rather than a failure of surgery.[7] Clinicians must be vigilant with respect to the natural history of osteoarthritis because the sequelae can compromise the efficacy of subsequent fusion procedures. Additionally, damage to the articular surface that could occur at the time of surgery may accelerate the rate of arthritic decline.[22] When the arthritic changes become severe enough, it could lead to decreased bone density and joint destruction, making subsequent arthrodesis more difficult and risky to perform.[23]

Scarring and Decreased Perfusion

As with any surgery, trauma from the exposure as well as the procedure itself can lead to soft tissue scarring and compromised vasculature, not only making a subsequent surgery more difficult to perform but also increasing the risk of complications.[24] Although first MTP joint fusion is a highly successful procedure with a generally low complication rates,[25–27] the effects from a prior cheilectomy may have a pronounced negative impact.

Complications

Acknowledging the potential for both intraoperative and postoperative complications during the index cheilectomy is a crucial consideration in treating hallux rigidus. Commonly encountered complications include the following:

- Overresection or underresection of the metatarsal head

- Soft tissue infection
- Osteomyelitis
- Delayed wound healing
- Avascular necrosis of the metatarsal head
- Chondrolysis
- Dorsal medial cutaneous nerve neuritis
- Malunion or nonunion from the Moberg osteotomy

Such complications, and their management, may further compromise the integrity of the first MTP joint. This can heighten the risk of complications during subsequent fusion.

BASELINE DEFICITS AFTER FAILED PRIMARY CHEILECTOMY

Cheilectomy is a highly successful procedure, frequently seeing more than 90% patient satisfaction for lower grades (grades I and II) and 85% satisfaction for higher grades (grade III).[1,4,28] Objectively, conversion to arthrodesis rates has been reported to be less than 10% within a decade after primary surgery.[15,29] Nevertheless, within this minority of cases that fail, patients may exhibit greater baseline functional impairments compared with those who have not undergone any prior surgical intervention when presenting for arthrodesis.

The first to evaluate the effects of prior cheilectomy on subsequent arthrodesis is a study by Rajan and colleagues, which demonstrated that among patients presenting for MTP joint fusion, individuals with a history of cheilectomy had inferior baseline physical function compared with the surgery-naïve cohort (PROMIS physical function score: 40.6 vs 44.4, $P = .028$).[30] It is difficult to propose a reason for this finding, and even more challenging to ascertain whether the diminished physical function stems from cheilectomy-related complications or failure, or due to the natural progression of arthritis. Equally challenging is accounting for the complex nature of patient expectations, which inherently introduces a subjective element difficult to control. Studies have shown that fulfillment of expectations, or lack thereof, is known to be correlated with postoperative patient-reported outcome scores.[31] Furthermore, the presence of complications after surgery, even if effectively addressed, could lead to unfulfilled expectations and further decrease patient-reported scores.[32,] Finally, given the vast majority of individuals achieve long-term satisfaction and seldom require reoperation after cheilectomy, the data may present an intrinsic sampling bias, emphasizing cheilectomy patients who did not fare well in contrast to naïve controls. Regardless, it seems that patients who present for MTP fusion after failed cheilectomy demonstrate inferior baseline function.

IMPROVEMENT AFTER METATARSOPHALANGEAL FUSION: PRIMARY VERSUS PRIOR CHEILECTOMY

Although patients who have undergone prior cheilectomy demonstrate worse baseline function compared with their counterparts when presenting for first MTP fusion, the success rate of the fusion is good. The aforementioned study illustrated similar improvements in all PROMIS domains across patient cohorts.[30] Despite initial functional limitations, MTP fusion results in commensurate clinical improvements, showing that patients may experience similar benefit from surgery. This attests to the efficacy of MTP fusion in preoperatively compromised patients and highlights its role as a viable salvage procedure following an unsuccessful cheilectomy. Consequently, surgeons can be encouraged to continue using cheilectomy as an initial surgical option with the comfort that, if required, a conversion arthrodesis can translate to a comparable magnitude of clinical benefit.

POSTOPERATIVE FUNCTION AFTER METATARSOPHALANGEAL FUSION: PRIMARY VERSUS PRIOR CHEILECTOMY

First MTP fusion has shown promising results, even when performed as a subsequent surgery after unsuccessful cheilectomy. Nonetheless, patients must still be counseled on postoperative expectations. Emerging data suggests that although the benefits from surgery are similar for patients postcheilectomy, their postoperative function is still inferior to those who underwent a primary fusion (PROMIS physical function 47.3 vs 51.2, $P = .017$).[30] This can be expected, as patients with a preceding cheilectomy tend to exhibit worse baseline function relative to their peers undergoing primary MTP fusion. Consequently, even with the surgery yielding consistent benefits across both groups, the postcheilectomy cohort retains suboptimal postoperative outcomes.

These findings neither invalidate the conversion procedure's efficacy nor preclude the need for salvage MTP fusion after failed cheilectomy. Rather, they provide more insight that can equip orthopedic surgeons for a preoperative dialog with patients that can better guide expectations.

COMPLICATIONS AFTER ARTHRODESIS

Complications following primary first MTP fusion remain relatively low, with the most common being nonunion and malunion. The nonunion rate is consistently under 10%, with some studies demonstrating a nonunion rate of 6.7% at an average of 47.3 months at the lower end and 8.6% at an average of 7.7 weeks at the higher end.[27,33] Similarly, the malunion rate has been reported to be around 6.1%, with an overwhelming majority being due to dorsal positioning of the hallux.[34] Other complications include interphalangeal joint arthritis, sesamoid pain, infection, and symptomatic hardware.

When comparing the complications between primary and conversion MTP fusions, data suggest similar complication rates. The only comparative study by Rajan and colleagues revealed a nonunion rate of 3.2% in the surgery-naïve group and 3.7% in those with history of prior cheilectomy, with no significant difference in the incidence ($P = .99$). The frequency of superficial infections was consistent between groups, with an incidence of 1.1% in the primary MTP fusion group and none in the prior cheilectomy group ($P = .99$). Similarly, the rate of hardware removal was similar, with 12.6% in the primary fusion group and 14.8% in the prior cheilectomy group ($P = .99$). The rates of postoperative interphalangeal joint pain, however, were different, with 1.1% of primary fusion patients experiencing adjacent joint pain compared with 11.1% of prior cheilectomy patients ($P = .034$).[30] Because these metrics are derived from a single study with a sample size of 122 feet, further research is warranted to better validate the difference in complication rates.

Should the clinician jump to primary fusion?

First MTP fusion is known to be the "gold standard" for definitively treating advanced stages of hallux rigidus (Hattrup and Johnson grade 3 or Coughlin and Shurnas grades 3 and 4).[15] The body of evidence surrounding the success of the procedure in these cases is robust, endorsing its use as a primary operation. However, cheilectomy has also established its merit, not only for treating milder stages but also for its efficacy in treating more advanced stages. O'Malley and colleagues demonstrated that when combined with a Moberg osteotomy for the treatment of Hattrup and Johnson grade III hallux rigidus, cheilectomy demonstrated favorable outcomes in more than 85% of patients, notably with only about 5% requiring conversion to arthrodesis.[4]

Recent literature has revealed comparable improvements in function and pain for patients who have previously undergone cheilectomy, with overall similar complication rates.[30] This suggests that although MTP fusion is a viable primary intervention, surgeons can also confidently use cheilectomy with Moberg osteotomy to address advanced stages of hallux rigidus, particularly if their patients are averse to any loss in great toe function. Further, because the literature reveals that only a minority of cheilectomy patients will go on to require conversion to MTP joint fusion even in more advanced stages, most patients will benefit initially with cheilectomy. Nonetheless, if cheilectomy fails, undergoing 2 surgeries can be challenging; therefore, for patients seeking the best chance to address their symptoms with a single procedure, MTP fusion is the preferred intervention. For early stages of hallux rigidus, cheilectomy with Moberg osteotomy remains the first-line treatment unless contraindicated because the success rate in these cases is even higher.

CONSIDERATIONS IN CHOOSING CHEILECTOMY VERSUS PRIMARY FUSION

Electing to perform a cheilectomy with or without Moberg osteotomy versus primary MTP fusion can have a few important considerations.

Patient-specific Health Factors

Comorbid medical conditions and patient age are key variables that influence the surgical decision-making process. The critical issue at hand is the likelihood of achieving successful fusion should the need arise. Because optimal arthrodesis is contingent on adequate bone stock and quality, among other factors, it is important that preexisting patient factors such as comorbidities and age be considered. Increased age, metabolic disorders such as diabetes and osteoporosis, and external variables such as exogenous steroid use have been identified as contributory risk factors for compromised union.[17,20,35,36] Therefore, in these high-risk patients, opting for a primary fusion before a cheilectomy could risk altering local factors such as bone stock and perfusion may be a judicious strategy. This approach would be geared toward ensuring the patient is best positioned to achieving a lasting, successful surgical outcome, even if a cheilectomy may otherwise be indicated.

Patient Expectations

Discerning patient expectations is a critical consideration when guiding patients on the most appropriate surgical intervention. Consequently, understanding a patient's surgical objectives is paramount to endorse a specific modality over another. Given the differing postoperative function associated with cheilectomy and fusion, it is important that the patient be prepared for their respective recovery.

Recovery

Accounting for the recovery time after surgery may be salient to some patients. Cheilectomy offers a markedly quicker recovery timeframe compared with fusion.[7,11,24,37] Because successful joint fusion demands good opposition of the bone edges without mechanical disturbance, it necessitates an extended recovery period with limited functional status and non–weight-bearing for most surgeons.[10,12,27] In scenarios where patients are constrained by time yet afflicted with severe pain, an initial strategy of cheilectomy may serve as a prudent first-line therapeutic approach. This allows for the future consideration of joint fusion once the patient may have more time, if the cheilectomy proves to be insufficient. Current literature reveals a high success rate associated with cheilectomy, as well as similar clinical benefits between primary and conversion arthrodesis.[1,3,4,7,30] Therefore, patients may confidently elect to undergo cheilectomy with the option of subsequent joint arthrodesis should the need arise.

INTRAOPERATIVE CONSIDERATIONS: PRIMARY VERSUS CONVERSION SURGERY

Conversion to arthrodesis after failed cheilectomy can present intraoperative challenges compared with a primary fusion.

Aberrant Anatomy

Cheilectomy changes the bony structure of the distal first metatarsal. This modification can alter landmarks traditionally used by surgeons. Because these reference points shift or become less discernible, the procedure may become more challenging to execute.

Scarring

Scarring resultant from prior cheilectomy plays a significant role in subsequent surgical planning and execution.

- Presence of adhesions and dense scar tissue can complicate the surgical approach and closure.
- Scarring may necessitate excess debridement.
- Increased risk of extensor hallucis longus (EHL) injury.
- Extended operative time increases the risk of postoperative complications.

In general, scarring makes conversion arthrodesis more technically challenging to perform compared with a primary procedure.

Decreased Bone Stock

As cheilectomy resects part of the articular surface of the metatarsal head, there is often decreased bone stock, which results in less surface area available for the fusion. This is accentuated if the resection was overly aggressive, resecting over a third of the joint surface.[22] To maintain as much bone stock as possible, surgeons might opt for alternate techniques such as using cup-and-cone reamers. This method could be favored over making flat cuts with a microsagittal saw because it involves less bony resection, potentially leading to not only a more successful fusion but also a greater preservation of first ray length to reduce the risk of developing transfer metatarsalgia.[21,38] In situations where bone stock is significantly reduced, it may be necessary to incorporate bone grafting to replace the defect and help augment the fusion. Bone graft for minor defects could be harvested from the calcaneus or proximal tibia, whereas larger defects could be filled with corticocancellous grafts taken from the anterior iliac crest.[10,19,22]

Bone Alignment

The extended orientation of the proximal phalanx following a Moberg osteotomy makes it more difficult to properly align with the metatarsal during arthrodesis, predisposing the first MTP joint to be fused in excess dorsiflexion (**Fig. 2**). Following a Moberg osteotomy, not only does the position make application of a dorsal plate more challenging but it could also further exacerbate the dorsiflexion when using a contoured plate. Consequently, some authors advocate for using a lag screw fixation to stabilize the joint in an appropriate alignment prior to applying the dorsal plate,

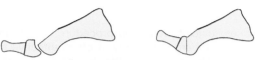

Fig. 2. Sketch depicting the risk of overdorsiflexing the proximal phalanx when performing a conversion MT fusion after failed cheilectomy with Moberg osteotomy.

which should be contoured by hand to better address the intrinsic dorsiflexion.[4] Care must be taken to properly angulate the proximal phalanx in about 10° to 15° of dorsiflexion to reduce the onset of metatarsalgia and painful interphalangeal joint callouses.[12,38] In some instances, bone grafting could be used to help rectify dorsal structural abnormalities and set the phalanx in a better position.[18]

FUTURE DIRECTIONS
Minimally Invasive Cheilectomy

More recently, minimally invasive (MIS) techniques have gained popularity due to their inherent advantages. The reduced surgical exposure translates to less soft tissue injury, decreased vascular compromise, and expedited patient recovery with less pain.[24,37] An increasing number of foot and ankle surgeons are receiving training in these techniques, leading to an increase in successful MIS cheilectomies. This could potentially improve the outcomes for patients undergoing conversion arthrodesis, given the reduced insult from the approach. Nonetheless, studies have shown a greater incidence of intra-articular debris retention within the MTP joint following MIS cheilectomy. Additionally, associated intra-articular pathologic conditions such as synovitis, loose chondral flaps, and loose bodies have been documented.[39,40] It will be important to compare the outcomes of MTP fusion patients who underwent prior MIS cheilectomy to those who underwent primary fusion. This could provide more insight into the efficacy of the MIS cheilectomy in relation to conversion arthrodesis.

CLINICS CARE POINTS

Electing to perform a cheilectomy or first MTP fusion requires careful evaluation of multiple factors including the potential for revision or conversion surgery. New research has provided more insight on the effect of prior cheilectomy on joint fusion, which can help guide decision-making. The following are some key points and takeaways:

- Cheilectomy and MTP joint fusion are performed with differing objectives and purposes; however, both are highly successful procedures for treating hallux rigidus.

- A cheilectomy does not preclude joint fusion; however, a joint fusion is definitive.

- Patients who have undergone prior cheilectomy demonstrate similar clinical improvements after MTP joint fusion compared with those who had primary fusion.

- Although prior cheilectomy does not affect the magnitude of improvement from MTP fusion, patients who have undergone cheilectomy have worse preoperative and postoperative function compared with those who have never undergone a prior procedure.

- Cheilectomy may be performed as a first-line option for more advanced stages of hallux rigidus without an increased risk for a failed subsequent fusion surgery compared with the inherent risk associated with primary arthrodesis.
  - However, patients must be counseled that they will likely have inferior postoperative outcomes compared with their counterparts.

SUMMARY

Cheilectomy is a successful joint-preserving procedure used to treat hallux rigidus. When augmented with a Moberg osteotomy, it offers effective treatment even for advanced disease stages. However, when the degeneration is severe enough, first MTP joint fusion remains the gold standard. Individualized patient evaluation and careful decision-making are essential for ensuring the most successful outcome for the patient. Clinicians may continue to use joint-preserving strategies in an attempt to maximize function and delay fusion because history of prior cheilectomy does not diminish the clinical benefits of conversion arthrodesis should the need arise. Nevertheless, patients must be counseled with clear postoperative expectations before proceeding with either surgery.

ACKNOWLEDGMENTS

We thank Dr Jaeyoung Kim for his expertise and assistance throughout all aspects of our study and for his help in writing the article.

DISCLOSURE

R Mizher, L Rajan, and J Kim have no disclosures. S J. Ellis receives consulting fees from Stryker, Paragon 28, Extremis, Medartis, Curvebeam, Extremity Medical, and Vilex in addition to serving as treasurer of the AOFAS foundation and on the editorial or governing board of Foot and Ankle Orthopedics.

REFERENCES

1. Coughlin MJ, Shurnas PS, Wilson S, et al. Hallux rigidus grading and long-term results of operative treatment. J Bone Joint Surg 2005;87(2):462–3.
2. Geldwert JJ, Rock GD, McGrath MP, et al. Cheilectomy : still a useful technique for grade I and grade II Hallux limitus/rigidus. J Foot Surg 1992;31(2):154–9.
3. Mackay DC, Blyth M, Rymaszewski LA. The role of cheilectomy in the treatment of hallux rigidus. J Foot Ankle Surg 1997;36(5):337–40.
4. O'Malley MJ, Basran HS, Gu Y, et al. Treatment of advanced stages of hallux rigidus with cheilectomy and phalangeal osteotomy. J Bone Joint Surg 2013;95(7): 606–10.
5. Vulcano E, Tracey JA3, Myerson MS. Accurate measurement of first metatarsophalangeal range of motion in patients with hallux rigidus. Foot Ankle Int 2016; 37(5):537–41.
6. Nawoczenski DA, Ketz J, Baumhauer JF. Dynamic kinematic and plantar pressure changes following cheilectomy for hallux rigidus: a mid-term followup. Foot Ankle Int 2008;29(3):265–72.
7. Easley ME, Davis WH, Anderson RB. Intermediate to long-term follow-up of medial-approach dorsal cheilectomy for hallux rigidus. Foot Ankle Int 1999; 20(3):147–52.
8. Kim PH, Chen X, Hillstrom H, et al. Moberg osteotomy shifts contact pressure plantarly in the first metatarsophalangeal joint in a biomechanical model. Foot Ankle Int 2015;37(1):96–101.
9. Henry JK, Kraszewski A, Volpert L, et al. Comparing first metatarsophalangeal joint flexibility in hallux rigidus patients pre- and postcheilectomy using a novel flexibility device. Foot & Ankle Orthopaedics 2020;5(2). 2473011420930000.
10. Koutsouradis P, Savvidou OD, Stamatis ED. Arthrodesis of the first metatarsophalangeal joint: The "when and how". World J Orthoped 2021;12(7):485–94.

11. Macklin Vadell A, Rofrano M, Bigatti A. Surgical treatment in hallux rigidus: dorsal cheilectomy and Moberg osteotomy. Journal of the Foot and Ankle 2022; 16(1):6–8.
12. Fuhrmann RA. First metatarsophalangeal arthrodesis for hallux rigidus. Foot Ankle Clin 2011;16(1):1–12.
13. Da Cunha RJ, MacMahon A, Jones MT, et al. Return to sports and physical activities after first metatarsophalangeal joint arthrodesis in young patients. Foot Ankle Int 2019;40(7):745–52.
14. Mann RA, Thompson FM. Arthrodesis of the first metatarsophalangeal joint for hallux valgus in rheumatoid arthritis. Journal of Joint and Bone Surgery 1984; 66(5):687–92.
15. Anderson MR, Ho BS, Baumhauer JF. Republication of current concepts review hallux rigidus. Foot and Ankle Orthopaedics 2023;8(3). 24730114231188123.
16. Napoli N, Chandran M, Pierroz DD, et al, IOF Bone and Diabetes Working Group. Mechanisms of diabetes mellitus-induced bone fragility. Nat Rev Endocrinol 2017;13(4):208–19.
17. Mitra R. Adverse effects of corticosteroids on bone metabolism: a review. PM & R 2011;3(5):466–71.
18. Grimm PD, Irwin TA. Complications of hallux rigidus surgery. Foot Ankle Clin 2022;27(2):253–69.
19. Khan SN, Cammisa FP, Sandhu HS, et al. The biology of bone grafting. J Am Acad Orthop Surg 2005;13(1):77–86.
20. Cruz A, Ropper AE, Xu DS, et al. Failure in lumbar spinal fusion and current management modalities. Semin Plast Surg 2021;35(01):54–62.
21. Winters BS, Czachor B, Raikin SM. Metatarsophalangeal fusion techniques with first metatarsal bone loss/defects. Foot Ankle Clin 2015;20(3):479–91.
22. Tomlinson M. Pain after cheilectomy of the first metatarsophalangeal joint. Foot Ankle Clin 2014;19(3):349–60.
23. Katz JN, Earp BE, Gomoll AH. Surgical management of osteoarthritis. Arthritis Care Res 2010;62(9):1220–8.
24. Stevens R, Burnsall M, Chadwick C, et al. Comparison of complication and reoperation rates for minimally invasive versus open cheilectomy of the first metatarsophalangeal joint. Foot Ankle Int 2020;41(1):31–6.
25. Doty J, Coughlin M, Hirose C, et al. Hallux metatarsophalangeal joint arthrodesis with a hybrid locking plate and a plantar neutralization screw. Foot Ankle Int 2013; 34(11):1535–40.
26. Goucher NR, Coughlin MJ. Hallux metatarsophalangeal joint arthrodesis using dome-shaped reamers and dorsal plate fixation: a prospective study. Foot Ankle Int 2006;27(11):869–76.
27. Chraim M, Bock P, Alrabai HM, et al. Long-term outcome of first metatarsophalangeal joint fusion in the treatment of severe hallux rigidus. Int Orthop 2016;40(11): 2401–8.
28. Sidon E, Rogero R, Bell T, et al. Long term follow-up of cheilectomy for treatment of hallux rigidus. Foot Ankle Int 2019;40(10):1114–21.
29. Roukis TS. The need for surgical revision after isolated cheilectomy for hallux rigidus: a systematic review. J Foot Ankle Surg 2010;49(5):465–70.
30. Rajan L, Kim J, An T, et al. Effect of prior cheilectomy on outcomes of first metatarsophalangeal joint fusion for treatment of hallux rigidus. Foot and Ankle Orthopaedics 2022;7(3). 24730114221119740.
31. Henry JK, Roney A, Cody EA, et al. Fulfillment of expectations after orthopedic foot and ankle surgery. Foot Ankle Int 2019;40(11):1249–59.

32. Chrea B, Day J, Henry J, et al. Influence of complications and revision surgery on fulfillment of expectations in foot and ankle surgery. Foot Ankle Int 2021;42(7): 859–66.

33. Kannan S, Bennett A, Chong HH, et al. A multicenter retrospective cohort study of first metatarsophalangeal joint arthrodesis. J Foot Ankle Surg 2021;60(3):436–9.

34. Roukis TS. Nonunion after arthrodesis of the first metatarsal-phalangeal joint: a systematic review. J Foot Ankle Surg 2011;50(6):710–3.

35. Filippi J, Briceno J. Complications after metatarsal osteotomies for hallux valgus. Foot Ankle Clin 2020;25(1):169–82.

36. Nicholson JA, Makaram N, Simpson A, et al. Fracture nonunion in long bones: A literature review of risk factors and surgical management. Injury 2021;52:S3–11.

37. Schipper ON, Day J, Ray GS, et al. Percutaneous techniques in orthopedic foot and ankle surgery. Orthop Clin N Am 2020;51(3):403–22.

38. Ho B, Baumhauer J. Hallux rigidus. EFORT Open Reviews 2017;2(1):13–20.

39. Glenn RL, Gonzalez TA, Peterson AB, et al. Minimally invasive dorsal cheilectomy and hallux metatarsal phalangeal joint arthroscopy for the treatment of hallux rigidus. Foot & Ankle Orthopaedics 2021;6(1). 2473011421993103.

40. Boffeli TJ, Collier RC, Thompson JC, et al. Cheilectomy combined with first tarsometatarsal joint arthrodesis for surgical treatment of midstage hallux rigidus complicated by medial column insufficiency: prospective evaluation of outcomes. J Foot Ankle Surg 2020;59(4):829–34.

Surgical Management of Failed First Metatarsophalangeal Joint Arthroplasty

Albert T. Anastasio, MD[a,1,*], Isabel Shaffrey, BS[b],
Mark E. Easley, MD[a,1]

KEYWORDS

- MTP joint • Metatarsophalangeal joint arthroplasty • Failed MTP joint arthroplasty
- Cartiva • Failed cartiva • MTP arthrodesis • Metatarsophalangeal joint arthrodesis

KEY POINTS

- Treatment of failed first metatarsophalangeal (MTP) joint arthroplasty can present a challenge to foot and ankle surgeons, and conservative measures often are unsuccessful.
- Conversion to arthrodesis of the MTP joint provides reliable joint stability while maintaining hallux length and reducing pain to the joint.
- Restoration of hallux length is of paramount importance in the treatment of failed MTP joint arthroplasty, and bony voids created by the removal of the MTP joint implant can be filled utilizing autograft, allograft, or metallic wedge implants.
- Maintaining appropriate dorsiflexion/plantarflexion positioning of the first MTP joint can prove challenging, and careful intraoperative attention to both clinical and radiographic appearance of the joint is imperative.

 Video content accompanies this article at http://www.foot.theclinics.com.

INTRODUCTION

Hallux rigidus is a prevalent, degenerative condition affecting the first metatarsophalangeal (MTP) joint. It is the most common form of arthritic disease in the foot, and is characterized by pain, restricted range of motion (ROM), and osteophyte formation. Substantial limitations in dorsiflexion can prove debilitating in afflicted patients, leading to altered gait mechanics and impaired ambulation.

[a] Department of Orthopaedics, Duke University Hospital, Durham, NC, USA; [b] Duke University School of Medicine, 2927 40 Duke Medicine Circle 124 Davison Building, Durham, NC 27710, USA
[1] Present address: 200 Trent Drive, Durham, NC 27710.
* Corresponding author. 200 Trent Drive, Durham, NC 27710.
E-mail address: Albert.anastasio@duke.edu

Foot Ankle Clin N Am 29 (2024) 541–556
https://doi.org/10.1016/j.fcl.2023.12.009
1083-7515/24/© 2023 Elsevier Inc. All rights reserved.

foot.theclinics.com

Management of hallux rigidus can pose a significant challenge to the treating provider. Though nonsurgical treatments should be attempted first, surgical management may be necessary in severe presentations of first MTP arthritis. Surgical interventions are variable and may be indicated based on degeneration severity and patient goals; these options include cheilectomy, first metatarsal osteotomy, resection arthroplasty, interpositional arthroplasty, implant arthroplasty, and hallux MTP joint arthrodesis.

In presentations of end-stage hallux rigidus, arthrodesis of the first MTP joint is the gold standard intervention for reliable pain relief and stability.[1] However, while arthrodesis has demonstrated consistently positive outcomes for pain and patient satisfaction, it also has been associated with symptomatic stiffness to the forefoot and midfoot and progressive adjacent joint arthritis. As such, arthroplasty of the first MTP joint has gained interest as a potential motion-sparing alternative to arthrodesis for hallux rigidus. Several variations of arthroplasty have been described for treatment of hallux rigidus, which range from total joint arthroplasty to hemiarthroplasty of the proximal phalanx or metatarsal and interpositional arthroplasty.[2,3] These techniques all typically involve cheilectomy, resection of one or both bony surfaces, and placement of an implant and/or biological spacer. Contrasted to MTP arthrodesis, arthroplasty of the first MTP joint optimally may offer preservation of ROM and improved function, while still eliminating or reducing pain in the joint.[3] In practice, success of the first MTP arthroplasty for treatment of hallux rigidus has been variable. Outcomes following interpositional arthroplasty have generally reported significant improvements in outcomes scores and ROM; however, high complication rates have also been reported.[4,5] Importantly, implant failure is associated with high rates of osteolysis and subsidence, creating large bony defects that can jeopardize the length and stability of the MTP joint. Thus, salvage options are limited, requiring robust fixation and substantial bone grafting to fill in osseous defects.[6,7]

While arthroplasty options for Hallux Rigidus (HR) may be successful, several series have reported high failure rates, necessitating revision surgery, often in the form of MTP joint arthrodesis. Given the high incidence of MTP arthroplasty procedures, the incidence of failed MTP arthroplasty is expected to increase over the coming decades. Thus, the purpose of this review is to discuss the surgical management of failed MTP arthroplasty, focusing primarily on MTP arthrodesis. Additionally, 2 cases of failure of different MTP joint arthroplasty devices will be presented, with in-depth discussion of surgical technique.

BACKGROUND ON METATARSOPHALANGEAL JOINT ARTHROPLASTY

Implant arthroplasty of the first MTP joint was first described in the 1970s, using a single-stemmed silastic implant. The initial version of this MTP implant was designed to preserve ROM and maintain the length of the hallux. However, early reports of the silastic implants described high rates of osteolysis and subsidence,[8,9] along with immunologic reaction to silicone debris that further accelerated joint degradation.[10–12] Salvage following failure of the silastic implant posed a significant challenge given the degree of osseous deficits, requiring substantial bone grafting during arthrodesis.[13] Use of the silastic implant for first MTP arthroplasty has since been limited in current practice.

Metallic hemiarthroplasty of the first MTP joint was developed as an alternative method to preserve joint movement. The design of the implant is intended as a replacement to the articular surface of the proximal phalanx or metatarsal head, while minimizing bone resection and implant debris. In general, outcomes of the metallic hemiarthroplasty for the MTP joint have been mixed; some authors have reported high rates of satisfaction and low incidence of revision,[14,15] while others cite high rates of failure.[16,17]

Modern generations of the first MTP arthroplasty have led to the introduction of a total toe arthroplasty featuring a metal-on-polyethylene implant design. These 3-component implants afford independent motion of the first MTP joint, with a cartilage-like interface between the 2 articulating surfaces. Though implant design has been modified and improved over time, the total toe arthroplasty has failed to show the consistent successful outcomes reported following MTP joint arthrodesis. Some authors have reported success with improved ROM and high patient satisfaction,[18] while others have reported high complication rates and incidence of early failure.[2,19] Current studies are limited to small cohorts and short follow-up periods, and thus the results remain inconclusive.

The polyvinyl alcohol (PVA) hydrogel implant (Cartiva, Stryker; Kalamazoo, MI) for MTP arthroplasty is a novel technology first introduced for use in the United States in 2016. This implant sits flush in the first metatarsal head and acts as a bumper between the 2 bony interfaces, both functioning as a hemiarthroplasty and interpositional arthroplasty. Composed of PVA hydrogel, the implant features several properties that mimic human cartilage, including high tensile strength, compressibility, and water content.[20] In a randomized study comparing results of PVA hydrogel implant versus arthrodesis, there were similar outcomes reported in terms of pain relief, function, and revision rates at 2 years.[21] However, other studies have demonstrated low satisfaction scores, high rates of reoperation, and early failures necessitating conversion to arthrodesis.[22,23] Though the PVA hydrogel implant may provide superior ROM and comparable pain relief, stability, and satisfaction when compared to arthrodesis, management following implant failure is difficult due to significant bone loss. Further long-term studies are needed to indicate its use.

CLINICAL PRESENTATION

Manifestations of failed MTP joint implant arthroplasty may present as localized pain, swelling, or redness near the first MTP joint. Patients may demonstrate reduced ROM and limited ambulation due to implant malposition, subsidence, or fracture. The most common cause of first MTP arthroplasty failure is due to progressive osteolysis, loosening, or fragmentation of surrounding bone, leading to subsidence of the MTP joint implant. It is imperative to screen for any symptoms of infection, including redness, swelling, wound drainage, and fever. If there is concern for infection, cultures should be taken intraoperatively, and antibiotics should be administered.

IMAGING

In patients who present with a surgical history of MTP arthroplasty and progressive pain, forefoot deformity, and swelling, standard radiographs and weightbearing films should be obtained. Radiographs of the foot are useful for assessing overall alignment, degree of bone loss at the MTP joint, and shortening of the first ray.[24,25] Computed tomography (CT) scanning can provide an accurate representation of the degree of bone loss present at the MTP joint.[26]

CT scan can also be used in the postoperative period after conversion to MTP arthrodesis to assess for bony union across the fusion site.[27] Weightbearing CT is emerging as a useful adjunct to provide information regarding the global alignment of the loaded foot.[28] MRI can be employed, but utility may be limited when compared to CT scan. The potential for metal artifact on MRI exists depending on the subtype of the index MTP arthroplasty and MRI may exhibit a decreased capacity to provide a more accurate representation of the degree of metatarsal bone loss.

TREATMENT

In patients who have been diagnosed with a failed MTP joint arthroplasty and present with symptoms of pain, instability, and swelling, various treatment options can be employed. These include nonoperative treatment modalities, as well as surgical options.

Conservative Treatment

Conservative treatment can be trialed in the setting of failed MTP arthroplasty. Chiefly, a supportive orthotic with a carbon fiber or steel shank may provide stability to the first ray and lead to symptomatic improvement.[29] Additionally, anti-inflammatory medications and activity modification can provide some relief, but represent poor long-term treatment options.[30]

Surgical Treatment

Surgical treatment is often required in the setting of failed MTP arthroplasty, as conservative options may provide only minimal relief in the setting of MTP joint instability, progressive bony erosion, and transfer metatarsalgia occurring due to a shortened first ray. While revision MTP arthroplasty can be considered in some circumstance, the gold standard for treatment of failed MTP arthroplasty remains MTP arthrodesis, either with or without block augmentation in the form of autograft, allograft, or synthetic materials.[24] The authors' preferred technique is described below for 2 separate cases: (1) Revision to MTP arthrodesis for failure of a metallic MTP arthroplasty implant, and (2) revision to MTP arthrodesis for failure of the PVA hydrogel implant.

EXPOSURE

The patient is brought to the operating theater and is positioned supine with fluoroscopy accessible throughout the procedure. A dorsomedial incision over the first MTP joint is made, optimally utilizing the previous surgical incision. Often, extension of the incision both distally and proximally will be required to adequately visualize the extent of bony erosion and appropriately position dorsal plating and other fixation modalities. The extensor hallucis longus tendon is mobilized and retracted laterally such that it may be carefully protected for the duration of the case. Furthermore, the dorsal medial cutaneous nerve, if identified, is carefully dissected and protected. Soft tissue dissection is carried to the level of the first MTP joint and a longitudinal capsular incision is made. Capsular tissue is then reflected to obtain exposure of the failed MTP arthroplasty device.

CASE I: REVISION TO METATARSOPHALANGEAL ARTHRODESIS FOR FAILURE OF A SILASTIC METATARSOPHALANGEAL ARTHROPLASTY IMPLANT

Anteroposterior and lateral radiographs of a patient presenting with continued pain to the right first MTP joint after a failure of a silastic MTP arthroplasty implant were obtained revealing implant subsidence (**Fig. 1**). The patient elected to undergo surgery. After exposure of the MTP join as outlined earlier, the silastic first MTP joint implant was dentified (**Fig. 2**). In this case, the components were noted to be loose and were easily extracted. Upon evaluation of the joint after component extraction, the relief areas within the MTP joint were eccentric, particularly in the metatarsal head. Thus,

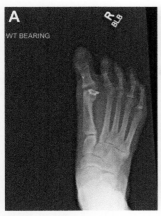
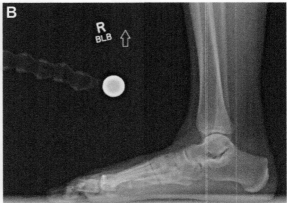

Fig. 1. (*A*) Anteroposterior (AP) and (*B*) lateral radiograph of a patient presenting with continued pain to the right first metatarsophalangeal (MTP) joint after a failure of a silastic MTP arthroplasty implant. The patient elected to undergo surgery.

these defects were curetted, removing all fibrous tissue. Subsequently, the defects were drilled to promote fusion and a bone graft mixture with orthobiologic adjuncts was packed into the joint defect.

After grafting of the defects, reaming was deemed to be feasible. With the soft tissues well protected, a dedicated reamer system was utilized to create a cup-and-cone preparation for the MTP joint. The surfaces were then drilled to promote successful arthrodesis. Given a significant shortening of the first MTP joint, a dedicated interpositional structural bone graft was sized and placed (**Fig. 3**). With the structural graft in place, the joint was reduced to an anatomic position and stabilized with provisional fixation utilizing a Kirschner (K)-wire. Optimal alignment and rotation were established, along with optimal bony apposition, and this was confirmed on fluoroscopy.

A compression screw was then placed from proximal medial to distal lateral, under fluoroscopic guidance. The screw was found to provide satisfactory compression and was confirmed to be in optimal position on fluoroscopy. Moreover, toe position was confirmed to be satisfactory utilizing a foot plate. Thus, final fixation was placed. To accomplish this, a dorsal plate was placed with satisfactory bone contact and was secured with screw fixation. Solid purchase of all screws in the bone was achieved prior to locking into the plate.

Intraoperative fluoroscopy confirmed satisfactory alignment of the first MTP joint and satisfactory bony apposition and positioning of the hardware. Rotation at the first MTP joint fusion site was evaluated both clinically and radiographically and was found to be appropriate. At this time, thorough irrigation was performed with copious amounts of sterile saline mixed with antibiotics and additional bone graft was packed at the arthrodesis site using bone excised from metatarsal head procedures done concomitantly for the lesser metatarsals through a separate incision.

The wounds were then closed in layers, with absorbable suture for the deeper layers including the capsular tissue for the MTP joint and the subcutaneous layers and nylon suture in an interrupted fashion to a tension-less closure without blanching at the skin bridges. Sterile dressings were placed over the wound and a splint was applied. The patient was non-weightbearing to the forefoot for 6 weeks, followed by a period of gradual weightbearing progression. Radiographs were obtained at post-operative follow-up visits and revealed excellent overall positioning of the forefoot and great

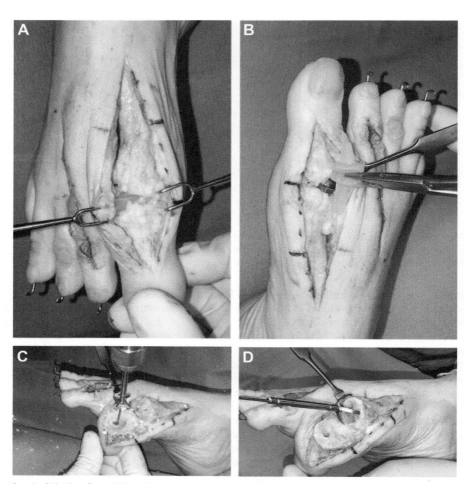

Fig. 2. (*A*) The first MTP joint was exposed, retracting the extensor hallucis longus (EHL) tendon laterally. (*B*) The polyvinyl alcohol (PVA) hydrogel implant was appreciated and the implant was found to be unstable and was easily removed. (*C*) After choice of appropriate reamer size, a dedicated reamer was used to ream the implant recipient site to freshen the defect in the metatarsal head to promote healing and to create a cup-and-cone preparation. (*D*) Finally, the proximal portion of the first toe phalanx was reamed using the dedicated reamer.

toe, with bridging bone at the arthrodesis site, and proper dorsiflexion/plantarflexion positioning of the great toe on lateral radiograph (**Fig. 4**).

CASE II: REVISION TO METATARSOPHALANGEAL ARTHRODESIS FOR FAILURE OF THE POLYVINYL ALCOHOL HYDROGEL IMPLANT

Anteroposterior and lateral radiographs of a patient presenting with continued pain to the right first MTP after a failure of the PVA hydrogel implant were obtained revealing graft subsidence and narrowing of the joint space (**Fig. 5**). The patient elected to proceed to surgery (Video 1). After exposure of the first MTP described earlier, deformity

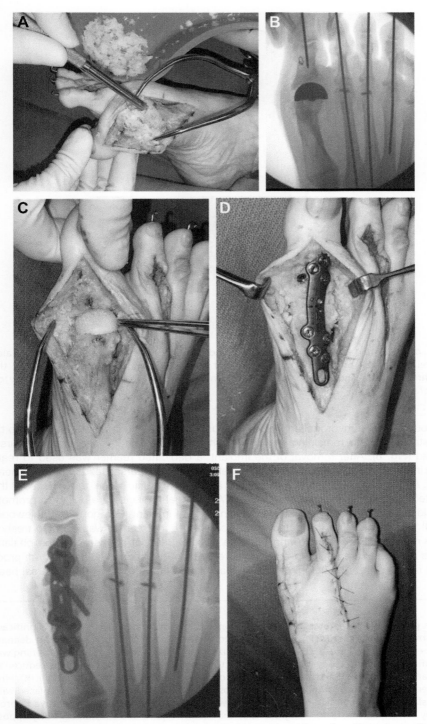

Fig. 3. (*A*) After thorough irrigation with copious amounts of sterile saline, the surfaces were drilled to promote fusion and a bone graft product mixed with orthobiologic adjuncts

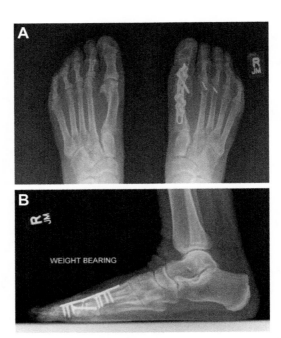

Fig. 4. (A) AP and (B) lateral weightbearing radiographic views at 1 year follow-up revealed excellent overall positioning of the forefoot and great toe, with bridging bone at the arthrodesis site, and proper dorsiflexion/plantarflexion positioning of the great toe on lateral radiograph.

through the PVA hydrogel implant was appreciated and the implant was found to be unstable, though remaining reduced in the space created in the first metatarsal head (**Fig. 6**). After removal of the implant, a dedicated reamer was used to ream the implant recipient site to freshen the defect in the metatarsal head to promote healing. After thorough irrigation with copious amounts of sterile saline, the surfaces at the defect created by the removal of the PVA hydrogel implant were drilled to promote fusion. Next, the AVITRAC MTP Revision System implant (Paragon 28; Englewood, CO) was placed into the defect and a cup-and-cone reamer was used to freshen the metatarsal head. Following this, the proximal aspect of the great toe phalanx was reamed to create a cup-and-cone preparation. Subsequently, a bone graft product mixed with orthobiologic adjuncts was placed in the remaining metatarsal head

was placed in the metatarsal head defect and at the arthrodesis site. Given a significant shortening of the first MTP joint, a dedicated interpositional structural bone graft deemed to be appropriate for use. This implant was sized and placed, and sizing and positioning was confirmed on fluoroscopy (B). With the structural graft in place (C), the joint was reduced to an anatomic position and stabilized with provisional fixation utilizing a Kirschner (K) wire. After placement of a compression screw across the MTP joint, a dorsal plate was placed with satisfactory bone contact and was secured with screw fixation (D). Intraoperative fluoroscopy confirmed satisfactory alignment of the first MTP joint and satisfactory bony apposition and positioning of the hardware (E). Finally, the wounds were closed in layers, and clinical evaluation of the forefoot revealed excellent overall alignment (F).

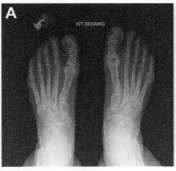 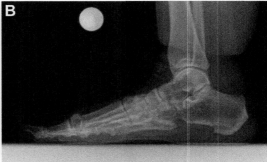

Fig. 5. (*A*) AP and (*B*) lateral radiograph of a patient presenting with continued pain to the right first MTP joint after a failure of the PVA hydrogel implant (Cartiva; Stryker, Kalamazoo, MI). The patient elected to undergo surgery.

defects and at the arthrodesis site. The joint was then reduced to an anatomic position and was stabilized utilizing a K-wire for provisional fixation. The reduction was confirmed on fluoroscopic imaging and overall simulated foot positioning in weight-bearing was assessed through use of a foot plate (**Fig. 7**).

A compression screw was then applied from medial-distal to lateral-proximal with satisfactory purchase. Following this, a neutralizing dorsal plate was placed and sequentially filled with multiple screws, with all screws having satisfactory purchase in bone prior to locking into the plate. Thorough irrigation was performed with copious amounts of sterile saline mixed with antibiotics and the wound was then closed in layers with absorbable suture for the deeper layers, including the capsular tissue for the MTP joint and the subcutaneous layers and nylon suture for the skin. Sterile dressings and a splint were applied, and satisfactory capillary refill was confirmed to remain in all the toes. The patient was non-weightbearing to the forefoot for 6 weeks, followed by a period of gradual weightbearing progression. Radiographs were obtained at post-operative follow-up visits and revealed excellent overall positioning of the forefoot and great toe, with clinical examination revealing proper forefoot weightbearing mechanics (**Fig. 8**).

OUTCOMES

Failure of first MTP implant arthroplasty is a challenging clinical scenario with limited salvage options. Significant deficits in available bone stock and shortening of the first ray following implant failure are predominate concerns in the revision setting that can complicate surgical planning. Arthrodesis of the first MTP joint is a reliable salvage procedure for the failed MTP arthroplasty that is effective in restoring first ray length and alignment.[1,31] It is a powerful tool that can be used in conjunction with grafting or synthetic wedge options to optimize the functionality and stability of a failed MTP joint arthroplasty procedure with significant osseous deficiencies.

Although outcomes following primary first MTP arthrodesis for hallux rigidus have been well described in the literature, results following salvage arthrodesis have not been consistently defined. In general, salvage arthrodesis for failed MTP implant arthroplasty can an effective, albeit imperfect, tool for the revision setting. Success rates of arthrodesis following first MTP implant arthroplasty have ranged between 80% and 100% in small cohort studies.[13,24,32–35] However, salvage arthrodesis has also demonstrated higher rates of nonunion, reoperations, and complications compared to primary

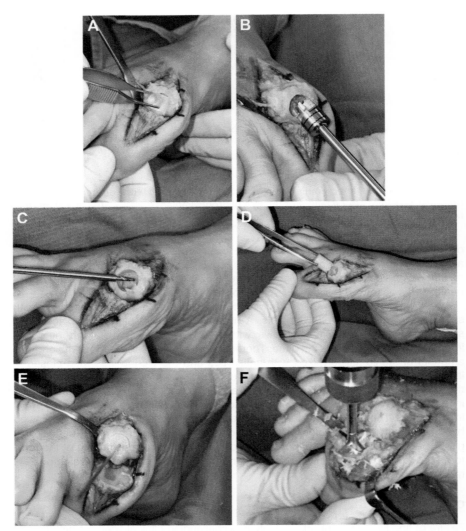

Fig. 6. After exposure of the first MTP, the PVA hydrogel implant was found to be unstable and was easily removed (*A*). A dedicated reamer was then used to prepare the implant recipient site to freshen the defect in the metatarsal head to promote healing (*B*). After thorough irrigation with copious amounts of sterile saline, the surfaces at the defect created by the removal of the PVA hydrogel implant were drilled to promote fusion (*C*). Next, the AVITRAC MTP Revision System implant (Paragon 28; Englewood, CO) was placed into the defect (*D*) and a K- wire was placed into the metatarsal head to facilitate reaming with the cup-and-cone reamer (*E*). Following this, the proximal aspect of the great toe phalanx was reamed to finalize the cup-and-cone preparation (*F*).

arthrodesis. In a recent systematic review of salvage arthrodesis for implant failure, the overall nonunion rate was 16.5% at mean 48.1 months.[6] In contrast, nonunion following primary arthrodesis occurred at a rate of 5.4%.[36] The disparity in nonunion rates between primary and salvage arthrodesis is a predictable consequence of the diminished bone stock available in the revision setting in addition to the further disruption of

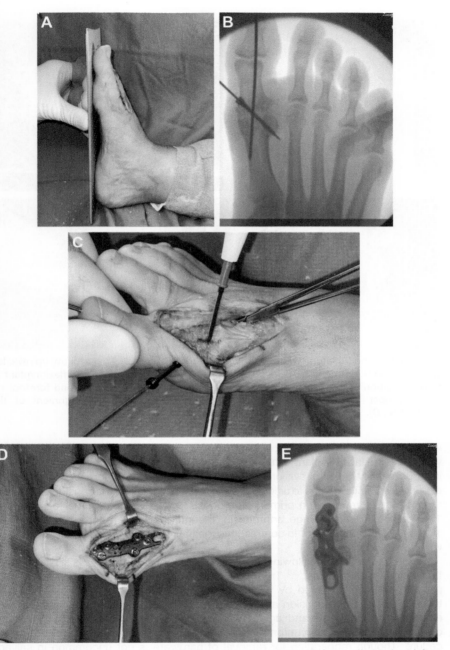

Fig. 7. The reduction was confirmed on fluoroscopic imaging and overall simulated foot positioning in weightbearing was assessed through use of a foot plate (*A*). A compression screw was then applied from medial-distal to lateral-proximal with satisfactory purchase (*B, C*). Following this, a neutralizing dorsal plate was placed and sequentially filled with multiple screws, with all screws having satisfactory purchase in bone prior to locking into the plate (*D*). Intraoperative fluoroscopic imaging confirmed appropriate alignment of the great toe and excellent positioning of the dorsal plate (*E*).

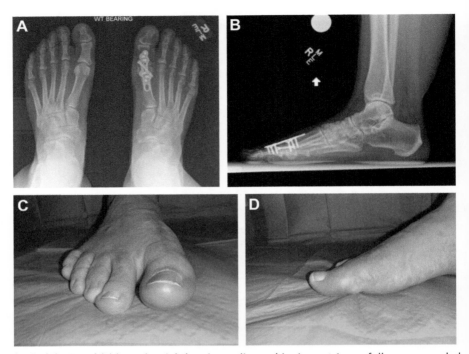

Fig. 8. (*A*) AP and (*B*) lateral weightbearing radiographic views at 1 year follow-up revealed excellent overall positioning of the forefoot and great toe and proper dorsiflexion/plantar-flexion positioning of the great toe. Clinical evaluation of the great toe and forefoot revealed proper positioning in weightbearing and excellent overall alignment of the forefoot (*C, D*).

vascular supply brought about by a secondary procedure. Bone resection and osteolysis due to the failed implant arthroplasty jeopardizes the structural integrity at the MTP joint, potentially causing revision arthrodesis to be challenging for surgeons with less experience. Similarly, time to union following revision arthrodesis is considerably higher than the rates reported in primary arthrodesis. Mean weighted time to union was 13 weeks following salvage arthrodesis, though individual reports range between 10.4 and 19.9 weeks.[6,13,24] In contrast, the mean time to union for primary arthrodesis was 9 weeks.[36]

Risk of complications following salvage first MTP joint arthrodesis is similarly higher than primary arthrodesis.[6,36] The most common complication following surgery is painful hardware, followed by wound dehiscence. To ensure sufficient stability of the MTP joint during revision arthrodesis, robust fixation is often necessary, often employing a dorsal plate and lag screw. Given the prominent profile of the hardware, development of pain is an unfortunate but common complication of the revision procedure. Though reoperation for removal of hardware is not uncommon in salvage arthrodesis,[13,24,34] it is imperative to ensure adequate healing is achieved before fixation is removed.

Fixation type and bone graft selection can have substantial impact on success of the revision arthrodesis procedure. During the salvage MTP joint arthrodesis, autologous or allogenic bone graft can be utilized to fill in osseous deficits. Iliac crest bone graft has been considered the gold-standard for bone graft options, despite reports of high comorbidities and complications.[37,38] In a systematic review of salvage arthrodesis following implant failure, the most frequently used bone graft was the iliac crest autograft (48%). Counterintuitively, the salvage MTP joint arthrodesis procedures which utilized iliac crest bone graft subsequently demonstrated the highest rate of nonunion (20%) relative to other forms of bone grating.[6] This incidence of nonunion with iliac crest autograft following salvage MTP joint arthrodesis is certainly higher than the rates described in the primary setting,[39] but in the salvage setting, the observed nonunion rates may be attributed to additional factors, such as surgeon choice to use iliac crest bone graft in cases involving more severe bony defects versus, for example, commercially available allograft wedges.

Ipsilateral calcaneal bone graft, morselized metatarsal head bone graft, and various types of allografts have also been utilized in the salvage setting with moderate success.[13,24,40] In a meta-analysis of salvage arthrodesis with or without bone graft, Mao and colleagues concluded there was fair evidence in support of arthrodesis with bone graft versus poor evidence to support arthrodesis without bone graft.[7] Despite high incidence of nonunion with MTP joint salvage arthrodesis, both with and without the use of bone graft, the literature generally points toward utilization of some form of bone graft as a necessary element to fill in osseous deficits following MTP arthroplasty implant failure.

Regarding clinical outcomes, the salvage MTP joint arthrodesis can successfully provide pain relief and has been correlated to improved function and patient satisfaction postoperatively. Garras and colleagues found that in a cohort of 18 patients who were revised from a failed hemiarthroplasty, visual analog scale pain scores diminished from 7.8 (out of 10) to 0.75 at final follow-up, while American Orthopedic Foot and Ankle Society function scores improved from 36.2 (out of 100) to 78.[35] These trends in diminished pain and improved function have been supported throughout several cohort studies of salvage arthrodesis following first MTP joint implant failure.[24,34] Furthermore, Usuelli and colleagues reported significant improvements in hallux valgus angle and 1 to 2 intermetatarsal angle without reduction in hallux length following arthrodesis in the setting of failed MTP joint arthroplasty.[34] Thus, the salvage arthrodesis demonstrates high degree of utility in improving function and providing pain relief without sacrifice to the integrity or stability of the great toe.

Compared to other revision procedures for failed implant arthroplasty, salvage arthrodesis of the metatarsophalangeal joint has demonstrated the most consistently reliable outcomes in terms of stability, pain reduction, and patient satisfaction. Following implant failure, a limited number of alternative revision procedures have been described, including revision hemiarthroplasty, excisional arthroplasty, and replacement with synthetic cartilage implant (SCI).[41,42] However, these studies are limited to anecdotal experience and the subsequent outcomes have not been well defined. In a comparison of revision arthrodesis versus SCI replacement for treatment of the failed SCI implant, the revision arthrodesis cohort demonstrated greater pain reduction at final follow-up.[41] Outcomes regarding replacement SCI following primary failure should further explored given the increasing popularity of the SCI implant for hallux rigidus. Ultimately, revision arthrodesis has the greatest evidence supporting its indication for the salvage of the failed MTP implant, providing joint stability while maintaining hallux length.

SUMMARY

Hallux rigidus is a common arthritic condition affecting the first MTP joint that can be treated with various surgical interventions. Though arthrodesis is the gold standard treatment for severe hallux rigidus, MTP joint arthroplasty has been utilized as a motion-sparing alternative option. Implant failure after MTP joint arthroplasty can present challenging surgical considerations, including large osseous defects and joint instability, which can make salvage options limited. Salvage MTP joint arthrodesis is the recommended intervention following MTP arthroplasty failure, as this procedure can provide reliable pain relief and stability to the first ray.

CLINICS CARE POINTS

- MTP joint arthroplasty has been utilized as a motion-sparing alternative for hallux rigidus, and failure of MTP joint arthroplasty can pose considerable challenge to the foot and ankle surgeon.

- CT scanning can provide an accurate representation of the degree of bone loss present at the MTP joint, which is imperative prior to salvage MTP arthrodesis procedures, such that appropriate graft or synthetic bony void filling materials can be made available.

- Careful intraoperative attention to both clinical and radiographic appearance of the first MTP joint is crucial, as maintaining appropriate dorsiflexion/plantarflexion positioning of the first MTP joint can prove challenging.

- Proximal versus distal positioning of the dorsal plate can greatly impact the final toe positioning, and surgeons should ensure maintenance of appropriate MTP joint reduction during final hardware placement.

DISCLOSURE

M.E. Easley: Exactech, Inc: IP royalties; Paid consultant; Paid presenter or speaker; Research support. IFFAS: Board or committee member. Journal of Bone and Joint Surgery - American: Editorial or governing board. Paragon28: Paid consultant; Paid presenter or speaker. Saunders/Mosby-Elsevier: Publishing royalties, financial or material support. Springer: Publishing royalties, financial or material support. Treace Medical: IP royalties; Paid consultant; Paid presenter or speaker. Wolters Kluwer Health - Lippincott Williams & Wilkins: Publishing royalties, financial or material support. A.T. Anastasio: QPIX Solutions – Paid consultant. I. Shaffrey has nothing to disclose.

SUPPLEMENTARY DATA

Supplementary data related to this article can be found online at https://doi.org/10.1016/j.fcl.2023.12.009.

REFERENCES

1. Hamilton GA, Ford LA, Patel S. First Metatarsophalangeal Joint Arthrodesis and Revision Arthrodesis. Clin Podiatr Med Surg 2009;26(3):459–73.
2. Horisberger M, Haeni D, Henninger HB, et al. Total Arthroplasty of the Metatarsophalangeal Joint of the Hallux. Foot Ankle Int 2016;37(7):755–65.
3. Sullivan MR. Hallux Rigidus: MTP Implant Arthroplasty. Foot Ankle Clin 2009; 14(1):33–42.
4. Anderson MR, Ho BS, Baumhauer JF. Current Concepts Review. Foot Ankle Orthop 2018;3(2). 247301141876446.
5. Cook E, Cook J, Rosenblum B, et al. Meta-analysis of First Metatarsophalangeal Joint Implant Arthroplasty. J Foot Ankle Surg 2009;48(2):180–90.

6. So E, Wilson M, Chu AK, et al. Incidence of Nonunion of the First Metatarsophalangeal Joint Arthrodesis After Failed Implant Arthroplasty: A Systematic Review. Foot Ankle Spec 2023. 193864002311693.
7. Mao DW, Zheng C, Amatullah NN, et al. Salvage arthrodesis for failed first metatarsophalangeal joint arthroplasty: A network meta-analysis. Foot Ankle Surg 2020;26(6):614–23.
8. Shereff MJ, Jahss MH. Complications of Silastic Implant Arthroplasty in the Hallux. Foot Ankle 1980;1(2):95–101.
9. Shankar NS. Silastic Single-Stem Implants in the Treatment of Hallux Rigidus. Foot Ankle Int 1995;16(8):487–91.
10. Sammarco GJ, Tabatowski K. Silicone Lymphadenopathy Associated with Failed Prosthesis of the Hallux: A Case Report and Literature Review. Foot Ankle 1992; 13(5):273–6.
11. McNearney T, Haque A, Wen J, et al. Inguinal lymph node foreign body granulomas after placement of a silicone rubber (Silflex) implant of the first metatarsophalangeal joint. J Rheumatol 1996;23(8):1449–52.
12. Freed JB. The increasing recognition of medullary lysis, cortical osteophytic proliferation, and fragmentation of implanted silicone polymer implants. J Foot Ankle Surg 1993;32(2):171–9. Availsble at: http://europepmc.org/abstract/MED/8391361.
13. Hecht PJ, Gibbons MJ, Wapner KL, et al. Arthrodesis of the First Metatarsophalangeal Joint to Salvage Failed Silicone Implant Arthroplasty. Foot Ankle Int 1997; 18(7):383–90.
14. Townley CO, Taranow WS. A Metallic Hemiarthroplasty Resurfacing Prosthesis for the Hallux Metatarsophalangeal Joint. Foot Ankle Int 1994;15(11):575–80.
15. Kline AJ, Hasselman CT. Resurfacing of the Metatarsal Head to Treat Advanced Hallux Rigidus. Foot Ankle Clin 2015;20(3):451–63.
16. Raikin SM, Ahmad J, Pour AE, et al. Comparison of arthrodesis and metallic hemiarthroplasty of the hallux metatarsophalangeal joint. J Bone Joint Surg Am 2007; 89(9):1979–85.
17. Anderson MR, Ho BS, Baumhauer JF. Republication of "Current Concepts Review: Hallux Rigidus". Foot Ankle Orthop 2023;8(3). 24730114231188124.
18. Koenig RD, Horwitz LR. The Biomet Total Toe System utilizing the koenig score: A five-year review. J Foot Ankle Surg 1996;35(1):23–6.
19. Pulavarti RS, McVie JL, Tulloch CJ. First Metatarsophalangeal Joint Replacement Using the Bio-Action Great Toe Implant: Intermediate Results. Foot Ankle Int 2005;26(12):1033–7.
20. Noguchi T, Yamamuro T, Oka M, et al. Poly(vinyl alcohol) hydrogel as an artificial articular cartilage: Evaluation of biocompatibility. J Appl Biomater 1991;2(2):101–7.
21. Baumhauer JF, Singh D, Glazebrook M, et al. Prospective, Randomized, Multicentered Clinical Trial Assessing Safety and Efficacy of a Synthetic Cartilage Implant Versus First Metatarsophalangeal Arthrodesis in Advanced Hallux Rigidus. Foot Ankle Int 2016;37(5):457–69.
22. Cassinelli SJ, Chen S, Charlton TP, et al. Early Outcomes and Complications of Synthetic Cartilage Implant for Treatment of Hallux Rigidus in the United States. Foot Ankle Int 2019;40(10):1140–8.
23. Smyth NA, Murawski CD, Hannon CP, et al. The Use of a Synthetic Cartilage Implant for Hallux Rigidus: A Systematic Review. Foot Ankle Spec 2021;14(4):366–71.
24. Gross CE, Hsu AR, Lin J, et al. Revision MTP Arthrodesis for Failed MTP Arthroplasty. Foot Ankle Spec 2013;6(6):471–8.
25. Wanivenhaus F, Espinosa N, Tscholl PM, et al. Quality of Early Union After First Metatarsophalangeal Joint Arthrodesis. J Foot Ankle Surg 2017;56(1):50–3.

26. Greisberg J. The Failed First Metatarsophalangeal Joint Implant Arthroplasty. Foot Ankle Clin 2014;19(3):343–8.
27. Adamson P, Janney C, Chen J, et al. First Metatarsal Phalangeal Joint Arthrodesis without the Use of Hardware after Failed Arthroplasty: A Case Report. J Orthop Case Rep 2021;11(1). https://doi.org/10.13107/jocr.2021.v11.i02.2028.
28. Mens MA, Bouman CMB, Dobbe JGG, et al. Metatarsophalangeal and interphalangeal joint angle measurements on weight-bearing CT images. Foot Ankle Surg 2023;29(7):538–43.
29. Colò G, Fusini F, Samaila EM, et al. The efficacy of shoe modifications and foot orthoses in treating patients with hallux rigidus: a comprehensive review of literature. Acta Biomed 2020;91(14-S):e2020016.
30. Mann RA. Disorders of the First Metatarsophalangeal Joint. J Am Acad Orthop Surg 1995;3(1):34–43.
31. Attia AK, Heier KA. First Metatarsophalangeal Arthrodesis for the Failed Hallux. Foot Ankle Clin 2022;27(4):723–44.
32. Myerson MS, Schon LC, McGuigan FX, et al. Result of Arthrodesis of the Hallux Metatarsophalangeal Joint Using Bone Graft for Restoration of Length. Foot Ankle Int 2000;21(4):297–306.
33. Brodsky JW, Ptaszek AJ, Morris SG. Salvage first MTP arthrodesis utilizing ICBG: clinical evaluation and outcome. Foot Ankle Int 2000;21(4):290–6.
34. Usuelli FG, Tamini J, Maccario C, et al. Bone-block arthrodesis procedure in failures of first metatarsophalangeal joint replacement. Foot Ankle Surg 2017;23(3):163–7.
35. Garras DN, Durinka JB, Bercik M, et al. Conversion Arthrodesis for Failed First Metatarsophalangeal Joint Hemiarthroplasty. Foot Ankle Int 2013;34(9):1227–32.
36. Roukis TS. Nonunion after Arthrodesis of the First Metatarsal-Phalangeal Joint: A Systematic Review. J Foot Ankle Surg 2011;50(6):710–3.
37. Boone DW. Complications of iliac crest graft and bone grafting alternatives in foot and ankle surgery. Foot Ankle Clin 2003;8(1):1–14.
38. Scheerlinck LME, Muradin MSM, van der Bilt A, et al. Donor Site Complications in Bone Grafting: Comparison of Iliac Crest, Calvarial, and Mandibular Ramus Bone. Int J Oral Maxillofac Implants 2013;28(1):222–7.
39. Mankovecky MR, Prissel MA, Roukis TS. Incidence of Nonunion of First Metatarsal–Phalangeal Joint Arthrodesis with Autogenous Iliac Crest Bone Graft after Failed Keller–Brandes Arthroplasty: A Systematic Review. J Foot Ankle Surg 2013;52(1):53–5.
40. Burke JE, Shi GG, Wilke BK, et al. Allograft Interposition Bone Graft for First Metatarsal Phalangeal Arthrodesis: Salvage After Bone Loss and Shortening of the First Ray. Foot Ankle Int 2021;42(8):969–75.
41. Chopra A, Fletcher AN, Madi NS, et al. Revision Surgery After Failed Index Synthetic Cartilage Implant Resurfacing for Hallux Rigidus: Single-Surgeon 5-Year Experience. Foot Ankle Spec 2023. https://doi.org/10.1177/19386400221147773. 193864002211477.
42. Anakwe RE, Middleton SD, Thomson CE, et al. Hemiarthroplasty augmented with bone graft for the failed hallux metatarsophalangeal Silastic® implant. Foot Ankle Surg 2011;17(3):e43–6.

Moving?

Make sure your subscription moves with you!

To notify us of your new address, find your **Clinics Account Number** (located on your mailing label above your name), and contact customer service at:

Email: journalscustomerservice-usa@elsevier.com

800-654-2452 (subscribers in the U.S. & Canada)
314-447-8871 (subscribers outside of the U.S. & Canada)

Fax number: 314-447-8029

Elsevier Health Sciences Division
Subscription Customer Service
3251 Riverport Lane
Maryland Heights, MO 63043

*To ensure uninterrupted delivery of your subscription, please notify us at least 4 weeks in advance of move.

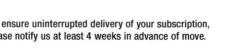

Printed and bound by CPI Group (UK) Ltd, Croydon, CR0 4YY

08/05/2025

01864748-0011